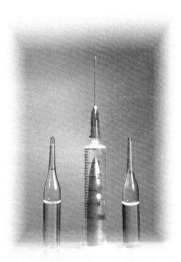

A MATHEMATICAL APPROACH
TO MULTILEVEL, MULTISCALE
HEALTH INTERVENTIONS

Pharmaceutical Industry Decline and Policy Response

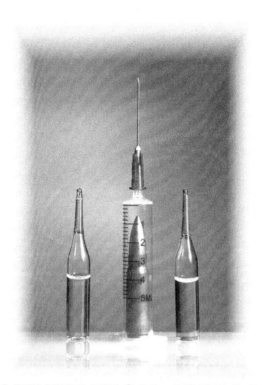

A MATHEMATICAL APPROACH TO MULTILEVEL, MULTISCALE HEALTH INTERVENTIONS

Pharmaceutical Industry Decline and Policy Response

Rodrick Wallace
Deborah Wallace

Columbia University, USA

Imperial College Press

Published by

Imperial College Press
57 Shelton Street
Covent Garden
London WC2H 9HE

Distributed by

World Scientific Publishing Co. Pte. Ltd.
5 Toh Tuck Link, Singapore 596224
USA office: 27 Warren Street, Suite 401-402, Hackensack, NJ 07601
UK office: 57 Shelton Street, Covent Garden, London WC2H 9HE

British Library Cataloguing-in-Publication Data
A catalogue record for this book is available from the British Library.

A MATHEMATICAL APPROACH TO MULTILEVEL, MULTISCALE HEALTH INTERVENTIONS
Pharmaceutical Industry Decline and Policy Response

ISBN 978-1-84816-996-8

Printed in Singapore by B & Jo Enterprise Pte Ltd

Preface

Many physiological phenomena involve the transmission of information. Even 'low level' regulatory processes, like gene expression and the operation of protein folding chaperones, can be interpreted as cognitive, in a formal sense, and associated with a 'dual' information source. Calculation shows that isolation of such sources from signal crosstalk between them consumes more metabolic free energy than does permitting correlation, allowing an evolutionary exaptation leading to dynamic global broadcasts of interacting physiological and larger cognitive modules at multiple scales and levels of organization. This is similar to the well-studied exaptation of noise to trigger stochastic resonance signal amplification.

The living state is therefore not only characterized by cognition at every scale and level, but by multiple, tunable, cooperative broadcasts that link selected subsets of modules to address problems facing the organism. This viewpoint has implications for current efforts in translational medicine that have followed the collapse of pharmaceutical industry magic bullet research. The central focus of such work is to speed the application of results available from laboratory studies at the molecular and cellular levels to drug development.

It is increasingly clear, however, that failure to respond to the inherently multilevel, multiscale nature of human pathophysiology dooms translational medicine: reductionist magic bullets are simply not enough. An essential feature of the full dynamic is that the principal environment for humans is other humans, their cultures, histories, and socioeconomic institutions – a layered composition of larger scale, interpenetrating cognitive and other structures and artifacts in which we all participate. Indeed, the evolutionary anthropologist Robert Boyd claims that culture is as much a part of human biology as the enamel on our teeth.

It is, then, necessary to seek, rather than reductionist magic bullets, carefully designed, synergistic, multilevel 'magic strategies' that will act across the scales and levels of organization of the human cognome – the overlapping assembly of cognitive modules within each human and the set of those in which each human is embedded – to restore normal function for individuals, populations, and even larger structures.

This book outlines a formal foundation for the design of such multilevel, multiscale treatment strategies, based on statistical models derived from the asymptotic limit theorems of information theory that provide a toolset for data analysis and policy construction. This work synthesizes, and significantly extends, a series of recently published papers, as listed below.

The material is presented at an advanced undergraduate mathematical level, assuming some knowledge of probability, abstract algebra, and calculus. Specialized topics are summarized in a Mathematical Appendix.

The most direct reading would be Chapters 1–3, followed by 10–12, with details filled in as needed from intermediate chapters that incorporate examples of the methodology.

The approach should be of compelling interest to the broad spectrum of scientifically informed policymakers who are called upon to pay the bill for increasingly expensive rearrangements of deck chairs on a reductionist biomedical *Titanic*.

Sources

Wallace, R., 2007, Culture and inattentional blindness: a global workspace perspective, Journal of Theoretical Biology, 245:378–390.

Wallace, R., 2008, Developmental disorders as pathological resilience domains, Ecology and Society, 13:29.

Wallace, R., 2010, Protein folding disorders: toward a basic biological paradigm, Journal of Theoretical Biology, 267:582–594.

Wallace, R., 2010, Expanding the modern synthesis, Comptes Rendus Biologies, 333:701–709.

Wallace, R., 2011, Structure and dynamics of the 'protein folding code' inferred using Tlusty's topological rate distortion approach, BioSystems, 103:18–26.

Wallace, R., 2011, Multifunction moonlighting and intrinsically disordered proteins: information catalysis, non-rigid molecule symmetries and the 'logic gate' spectrum, Comptes Rendus Chimie, 14:1117–1121.

Wallace, R., 2012, Extending Tlusty's rate distortion index theorem method to the glycome: Do even 'low level' biochemical phenomena require sophisticated cognitive paradigms? BioSystems, 107:145–152.

Wallace, R., 2012, Spontaneous symmetry breaking in a non-rigid molecule approach to intrinsically disordered proteins, Molecular BioSystems, 8:374–377.

Wallace, R., 2012, Consciousness, crosstalk, and the mereological fallacy: an evolutionary perspective, Physics of Life Reviews, doi 10.1016/j.plrev.2012.08.002.

Wallace, R., 2012, Metabolic constraints on the evolution of genetic codes: did multiple 'preaerobic' ecosystem transitions entrain richer dialects via Serial Endosymbiosis? Transactions on Computational Systems Biology XIV, LNBI 7625:204–232.

Wallace, R., D. Wallace, 2008, Punctuated equilibrium in statistical models of generalized coevolutionary resilience: how sudden ecosystem transitions can entrain both phenotype expression and Darwinian selection, Transactions on Computational Systems Biology IX, LNBI 5121:23–85.

Wallace, R., D. Wallace, 2009, Code, context, and epigenetic catalysis in gene expression, Transactions on Computational Systems Biology XI, LNBI 5750, 283–334.

Wallace, R., D. Wallace, 2011, Cultural epigenetics: on the heritability of complex diseases, Transactions on Computational Systems Biology XIII, LNBI 6575:131–170.

Wallace, R.G., R. Wallace, 2009, Evolutionary radiation and the spectrum of consciousness, Consciousness and Cognition, 18:160–167.

Contents

Preface   v

1. BEYOND MAGIC BULLETS   1

    1.1   The Pharmaceutical Catastrophe   1

    1.2   A New Perspective   6

    1.3   Cognition as 'Language'   8

    1.4   The Human Cognome   11

2. EXPANDING THE THEORY   19

    2.1   No Free Lunch   19

    2.2   Multiple Broadcasts, Punctuated Detection 22

    2.3   Metabolic Constraints   25

    2.4   Environmental Signals   27

3. DYNAMIC 'REGRESSION' MODELS   29

    3.1   The Simplest Approach   29

    3.2   A Rate Distortion Reformulation 35

    3.3   Multiple Time Scales   38

    3.4   Incoming Information   39

    3.5   Pathologies   40

    3.6   Refining the Model   42

4. AN EVOLUTIONARY EXCURSION   47

    4.1   Introduction   47

    4.2   Ecosystems as Information Sources 50

    4.3   Genetic Heritage   53

4.4   Gene Expression   54
4.5   Interacting Information Sources   56
4.6   Conclusions   59

5. EXAMPLE: MENTAL DISORDERS   63

5.1   Introduction   63
5.2   Two Classes   67
5.3   Global Broadcast Models   70
5.4   Gene Expression   72
5.5   Summary   74

6. EXAMPLE: PROTEIN FOLDING   77

6.1   Introduction   77
6.2   Spontaneous Symmetry Breaking   81
6.3   A Formal Approach   83
6.4   The Energy Picture   86
6.5   The Developmental Picture   86
6.6   A Comprehensive Treatment   91
6.7   Aging and Protein Folding   95
6.8   Summary   97

7. EXAMPLE: GLYCOME DETERMINANTS   99

7.1   Introduction   99
7.2   Stochastic Topology 101
7.3   The Glycomic Conundrum 103
7.4   Another Cognitive Paradigm 104
7.5   Regulating Glycan Determinants 108
7.6   Glycan Spectra 109
7.7   Summary 111

8. EXAMPLE: GLYCAN/LECTIN LOGIC GATES   113

8.1   Introduction 113
8.2   The Critical Exponent 114
8.3   Two Examples 116
8.4   Information Catalysis 120
8.5   A Tiling Symmetry Model 122
8.6   Summary 126

9. EXAMPLE: IDP LOGIC GATES 127

    9.1   Introduction 127

    9.2   Symbolic Dynamics of Molecular Switching 130

    9.3   Another Dual Information Source 131

    9.4   Information Catalysis 133

    9.5   Summary 134

10. TREATMENT 137

    10.1   The Generalized Retina 137

    10.2   Therapeutic Efficacy 141

    10.3   Psychosocial Stress 144

    10.4   Flight, Fight, and Helplessness 146

    10.5   Institutions as Niche Construction 148

    10.6   The Hall of Mirrors 150

    10.7   Side Effects Reconsidered 152

11. HISTORY AND HEALTH 157

    11.1   Malaria and the Fulani 157

    11.2   The American Catastrophe 160

12. BEYOND GLASPERLENSPIEL 179

13. MATHEMATICAL APPENDIX 183

    13.1   The Tuning Theorem 183

    13.2   The Rate Distortion Theorem 187

    13.3   Stochastic Differential Equations 189

    13.4   Morse Theory 194

    13.5   Groupoids 196

    13.6   'Biological' Renormalization 199

    13.7   Large Deviations 204

Bibliography 207

Index 223

Chapter 1

BEYOND MAGIC BULLETS

1.1 The Pharmaceutical Catastrophe

Pharmaceutical industry research productivity has collapsed. Figure 1.1, adapted from Bernstein (2010), shows the number of small molecule and biologic USFDA approvals per inflation-adjusted billion dollars in research investment between 1950 and 2010. The cost per 'magic bullet' has increased exponentially from about $200 million to over $1.2 billion, and many pharmaceutical firms have markedly cut their research efforts as a consequence of this 'inverse Moore's Law' that represents the failure of complex physiological phenomena to respond to simple, decontextualized, interventions.

Paul *et al.* (2010) summarize the crisis as follows:

> [W]ithout a dramatic increase in [Research and Development] productivity, today's pharmaceutical industry cannot sustain sufficient innovation to replace the loss of revenues due to patent expirations for successful products... [However]... a more complete understanding of human (disease) biology will... be required before many true breakthrough medicines emerge.

This dynamic has spawned attempts to speed the 'bench to bedside' translation of basic research into therapeutic instruments, usually seen as new magic bullets, drugs or otherwise.

In the words of the publisher of the recent volume by Littman and Krishna (2011), translational medicine

> ...seeks to translate biological and molecular knowledge of disease and how drugs work into innovative strategies

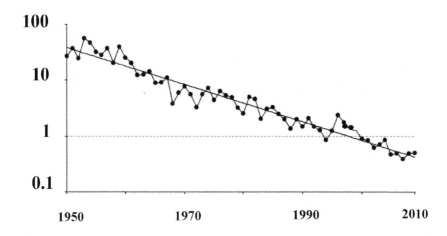

Fig. 1.1   Adapted from Bernstein (2010). The inverse Moore's Law for pharmaceuticals. The number of small molecule and biological USFDA approvals per inflation-adjusted \$ billion in research investment, 1950–2010. The apparent log-linear 'decline in research productivity' represents the failure of complex physiological phenomena to respond to simple interventions. Western medicine, as defined in the latter half of the 20th century, has hit a brick wall, a catastrophic regime of exponential cost increase.

that reduce the cost and increase the speed of delivering new medicines for patients.

Marincola (2011) has responded to current efforts with a scathing critique:

> Translational research is caught in a feedback cycle whereby complex, multi-factorial disease is confronted without sufficient understanding of human pathophysiology... It has been suggested that preclinical models do not represent human disease because of differences among species... However, this is not the principal reason they often fail to provide suitable models of human disease; the fundamental difference between preclinical and clinical testing is that in the former, the researcher can carefully select the model, whereas in the latter the clinician has to confront the unpredictable nature of human genetics and diseases, as well as environmental factors.

Wehling (2011) is more direct:

Approximately a decade ago, translational medicine was invented both as a catchword and as a novel approach to improve success in drug development and ameliorate the low-output syndrome from collapsing pipelines. However, no major breakthroughs regarding rates of expensive late attrition or market approvals have been detected, and drug industry condensation continues to accelerate... [T]ranslational efforts so far seem to be driven mainly by claims, rather than by structure and systematic approaches. In addition, institutional structures also often seem to be only virtual or proclaiming in nature. This is simply not enough.

Horrobin (2003) lays out the lack of congruence between laboratory-level *in vitro* and patient-level *in vivo* models:

An important distinction must be made between what might be called the anatomical biochemistry of the cell and its functional biochemistry... [I]f a particular biochemical step is present *in vitro*, then that particular biochemical step is also likely to be present... *in vivo*. We can therefore construct a network of all possible biochemical events *in vivo* by examining all possible biochemical events *in vitro*. But what the *in vitro* system cannot do is construct a functional and valid *in vivo* biochemistry. And that is potentially a fatal flaw. For in most human diseases it is the functional biochemistry and not the anatomical biochemistry which goes wrong.

Horrobin provides details, and we summarize his Table 1:

In Vitro vs. *In Vivo* models

1. The anatomical constraints and the cellular populations present in culture and *in vivo* are different. There is no circulation *in vitro*.
2. The types and rates of nutrient and oxygen supply, and carbon dioxide and metabolite removal, are different.
3. The restraints on cell multiplication are different.

4. The endocrine environment is different, both in terms of the amounts and patterns of hormones present and their kinetic changes.
5. The antibiotic environment is different: *in vivo* cells are not normally bathed in penicillin, streptomycin and other antibiotics, but there has been no systematic evaluation of the effects of any of these exogenous agents on metabolism.
6. The lipid environment is different. The phospholipid composition of cells in culture is quite different from the phospholipid composition of the parent *in vivo* cells. As phospholipid composition determines the quaternary structure and therefore function of a high proportion of a cell's proteins, and also determines signal transduction responses to most protein changes, it is likely that the functions of proteins *in vitro* will be, for the most part, somewhat different from the functions of those same proteins *in vivo*.
7. Even when appropriate constituents are present in culture fluid, their concentrations may be dramatically different from anything seen *in vivo*.

Horrobin (2003) goes on to liken current reductionist biomedicine to Herman Hesse's *Glasperlenspiel*, a Glass Bead Game, in which troublesome intellectuals have been seduced from real-world problems into an elaborate, heavily subsidized glass cage, lucrative for those who become skilled at grantsmanship.

Begley and Ellis (2012) provide a later case history. They report on attempts to reproduce the results of 53 'landmark studies' in preclinical cancer research. Six were reproducible.

They write:

Some non-reproducible preclinical papers had spawned an entire field, with hundreds of secondary publications that expanded on elements of the original observation, but did not actually seek to confirm or falsify its fundamental basis. More troubling, some of the research has triggered a series of clinical studies – suggesting that many patients had subjected themselves to a trial of a regimen or agent that probably wouldn't work...

Begley and Ellis recapitulate something of Horrobin's central observations contrasting *in vitro* with *in vivo* results:

The limitations of preclinical cancer models have been widely reviewed and are largely acknowledged by the field. They include the use of small numbers of poorly characterized tumor cell lines that inadequately recapitulate human disease, an inability to capture the human tumor environment, a poor appreciation of pharmacokinetics and pharmacodynamics, and the use of problematic endpoints and testing strategies...

Begley and Ellis, in their way, even recapitulate Horrobin's *Glasperlenspiel* assertion:

What reasons underlie the publication of erroneous, selective or irreproducible data? The academic system and peer-review process tolerates and perhaps even inadvertently encourages such conduct. To obtain funding, a job, promotion or tenure, researchers need a strong publication record, often including first-authored high-impact publication. Journal editors, reviewers and grant-review committees often look for a scientific finding that is simple, clear and complete – a 'perfect' story. It is therefore tempting for investigators to submit selected data sets for publication, or even to massage data to fit the underlying hypothesis.

But there are no perfect stories in biology.

The failure to reproduce preclinical cancer research has been mirrored, in a sense, by much larger – indeed, spectacular – failures of drugs actually marketed to perform as advertised. A *New York Times* Business Section story by Thomas (2012) describes a number of massive legal and regulatory penalties assessed against major pharmaceutical companies, as summarized below.

Company	Drug	Penalty ($ billion)
GlaxoSmithKline	Avandia	3.0
Pfizer	Bextra	2.3
Abbott Labs	Depakote	1.6
Eli Lilly	Zyprexa	1.4
J. and J.	Risperdal	1.2

In some contrast to current biomedical 'magic bullet' ideology – and its associated *Glasperlenspiel* and consumer fraud – this volume will attempt to lay a foundation for the development of multilevel, multiscale 'magic strategies' that may, at least in their initial stages, better fit the inherently complex underlying patterns of multifactorial human pathophysiology and its inherently imperfect biological story.

This is not an effort for the faint of heart, and it must begin far afield.

1.2   A New Perspective

Researchers have long speculated and experimented on the role of noise in biological process via models of stochastic resonance (e.g., Park and Nee-lakanta, 1996; Gluckman *et al.*, 1996; Ward, 2009; Kawaguchi *et al.*, 2011). The necessary ubiquity of noise affecting information transmission under-went an evolutionary exaptation (e.g., Gould, 2002) to become a tool for amplification of weak signals and, according to current thinking, a tool for cellular decision making. Balazsi *et al.* (2011) examine a cascade of cellular decision phenomena from viral to multiple-cellular levels of organization in terms of noise. They write:

> A growing number of cell types are being described as capable of decision making under various circumstances, suggesting that such cellular choices are widespread in all organisms... [Many such bio-logical] choices... may, in general, be stochastic, driven by random molecular noise within networks characterized by bistable or excitable dynamics. This hints at the possibility that some of the most stud-ied cellular processes... may be based on stochastic decision making inherited from ancient bimolecular circuits... The outcome of these stochastic decisions is an environment-dependent balance... There-fore, cellular decision making constitutes a very simple mechanism for pattern formation that does not require cell-cell interactions or intercell communication and can therefore operate from the lowest to the highest levels of biological complexity...

They caution, however:

> [E]xamples from mammalian cells indicate that cellular decision making underlies the most basic cellular processes in some of the most complex organisms, relying on regulatory networks with dynamics similar to those found in lower metazoans and microbes. However, the exact structure of the regulatory mechanisms controlling mam-

malian cell decisions is much less understood than for lower organisms... Moreover, the studies [we describe] were conducted in cell lines, and not actual mammals, and very little is known about mammalian cell fate choices *in vivo*.

Here, we attempt to move up in both scale and level of organization, from subcellular and cellular, to tissue, organism, and social structure. The central focus will be on the parallel necessary circumstance to 'noise', i.e., of information leakage between adjacent communication channels or information sources. This is a generally unwelcome signal correlation that the electrical engineers call 'crosstalk'. It is known to grow roughly as the inverse square of the distance between circuits, and is thus likely to be significant at molecular and cellular scales (Paul, 1992; Kuo *et al.*, 2007).

To cut to the chase, the evolutionary exaptation of crosstalk appears to be nested systems of shifting, global biological broadcasts analogous to, but both slower and more general than, animal consciousness.

Much theoretical work has already been done in this direction, using statistical tools constructed using the asymptotic limit theorems of information theory, a close analogy to parametric statistics constructed from the central limit theorem. The material appears adaptable to the design of multilevel health interventions. Some general background follows.

Baars' global workspace model of consciousness attributes the phenomenon to a dynamic array of unconscious cognitive modules that unite to become a global broadcast having a tunable perception threshold not unlike a theater spotlight, but whose range of attention is constrained by embedding contexts (e.g., Baars, 1988, 2005; Baars and Franklin, 2003):

1. The brain can be viewed as a collection of distributed specialized networks (processors).

2. Consciousness is associated with a global workspace in the brain – a fleeting memory capacity whose focal contents are widely distributed – 'broadcast' – to many unconscious specialized networks.

3. Conversely, a global workspace can also serve to integrate many competing and cooperating input networks.

4. Some unconscious networks, called contexts, shape conscious contents, for example unconscious parietal maps modulate visual feature cells that underlie the perception of color in the ventral stream.

5. Such contexts work together jointly to constrain conscious events.

6. Motives and emotions can be viewed as goal contexts.

7. Executive functions work as hierarchies of goal contexts.

The basic mechanism emerges 'naturally' from a relatively simple application of the asymptotic limit theorems of information theory, once a broad range of unconscious cognitive processes is recognized as inherently characterized by information sources – generalized languages (Wallace, 2000, 2005, 2007). The approach allows mapping physiological unconscious cognitive modules onto an abstract network of interacting information sources. This, in turn, permits a simplified mathematical attack based on phase transitions in network topology that, in the presence of sufficient linkage – crosstalk – permits rapid, shifting, global broadcasts.

While the mathematical description of consciousness is itself relatively simple, the evolutionary trajectories leading to its emergence seem otherwise. Here, we argue that this is not the case, and that physical restrictions on the availability of metabolic free energy provide sufficient conditions for the emergence, not only of consciousness, but of a spectrum of analogous 'global' broadcast phenomena acting across a variety of biological scales of space, time, and levels of organization.

The argument is, in a sense, an extension of Gould and Lewontin's (1979) famous essay "The Spandrels of San Marco and the Panglossian Paradigm: A Critique of the Adaptationist Programme". Spandrels are the triangular sectors of the intersecting arches that support a cathedral roof. They are simple by-products of the need for arches, and their occurrence is in no way fundamental to the construction of a cathedral. Our assertion is that crosstalk between 'low level' cognitive biological modules is a similar inessential by-product that evolutionary process has exapted to construct the dynamic global broadcasts of consciousness and a spectrum of roughly analogous physiological phenomena: evolution built many new arches from a single spandrel.

We provide a minimal formal overview that will be reexpressed in more complex form, much like Onsager's nonequilibrium thermodynamics, leading to 'dynamical' regression models that, in addition to providing new conceptual perspectives, should be useful in data analysis.

1.3   Cognition as 'Language'

Atlan and Cohen (1998) argue that, in the context of a cognitive paradigm for the immune system, the essence of cognitive function involves comparison of a perceived signal with an internal, learned or inherited picture of the world, and then, upon that comparison, choice of one response from a much larger repertoire of possible responses. That is, cognitive pattern recognition-and-response proceeds by an algorithmic combination of an incoming external sensory signal with an internal ongoing activity – incorporating the internalized picture of the world – and triggering an appropriate action based on a decision that the pattern of sensory activity requires a response.

More formally, incoming sensory input is mixed in an unspecified but systematic manner with a pattern of internal ongoing activity to create a path of combined signals $x = (a_0, a_1, ..., a_n, ...)$. Each a_k thus represents some functional composition of the internal and the external. An application of this perspective to a standard neural network is given in Wallace (2005, p. 34).

This path is fed into a highly nonlinear, but otherwise similarly unspecified, decision function, h, which generates an output $h(x)$ that is an element of one of two disjoint sets B_0 and B_1 of possible system responses. Let

$$B_0 \equiv \{b_0, ..., b_k\},$$

$$B_1 \equiv \{b_{k+1}, ..., b_m\}.$$

Assume a graded response, supposing that if

$$h(x) \in B_0,$$

the pattern is not recognized, and if

$$h(x) \in B_1,$$

the pattern is recognized, and some action $b_j, k+1 \leq j \leq m$ takes place.

The principal objects of formal interest are paths x which trigger pattern recognition-and-response. That is, given a fixed initial state a_0, we examine all possible subsequent paths x beginning with a_0 and leading to the event $h(x) \in B_1$. Thus $h(a_0, ..., a_j) \in B_0$ for all $0 \leq j < m$, but $h(a_0, ..., a_m) \in B_1$.

For each positive integer n, let $N(n)$ be the number of high probability grammatical and syntactical paths of length n that begin with some particular a_0 and lead to the condition $h(x) \in B_1$. Call such paths 'meaningful', assuming, not unreasonably, that $N(n)$ will be considerably less than the number of all possible paths of length n leading from a_0 to the condition $h(x) \in B_1$.

While combining algorithm, the form of the function h, and the details of grammar and syntax, are all unspecified in this model, the critical assumption permitting inference on necessary conditions constrained by the asymptotic limit theorems of information theory is that the finite limit

$$H \equiv \lim_{n \to \infty} \frac{\log[N(n)]}{n} \tag{1.1}$$

both exists and is independent of the path x.

Call such a pattern recognition-and-response cognitive process *ergodic*. Not all cognitive processes are likely to be ergodic, implying that H, if it indeed exists at all, is path dependent, although extension to nearly ergodic processes, in a certain sense, seems possible (e.g., Wallace, 2005, pp. 31–32).

Invoking the spirit of the Shannon–McMillan theorem, it is possible to define an adiabatically, piecewise stationary, ergodic information source **X** associated with stochastic variates X_j having joint and conditional probabilities $P(a_0, ..., a_n)$ and $P(a_n | a_0, ..., a_{n-1})$ such that appropriate joint and conditional Shannon uncertainties satisfy the classic relations (Cover and Thomas, 2006)

$$H[\mathbf{X}] = \lim_{n \to \infty} \frac{\log[N(n)]}{n} = \lim_{n \to \infty} H(X_n | X_0, ..., X_{n-1}) = \lim_{n \to \infty} \frac{H(X_0, ..., X_n)}{n}. \tag{1.2}$$

This information source is defined as *dual* to the underlying ergodic cognitive process, in the sense of Wallace (2000, 2005).

The essence of 'adiabatic' is that, when the information source is parameterized according to some appropriate scheme, within continuous 'pieces', changes in parameter values take place slowly enough so that the information source remains as close to stationary and ergodic as needed to make the fundamental limit theorems work. 'Stationary' means that probabilities do not change in time, and by 'ergodic' (roughly) that cross-sectional means converge to long-time averages. Between 'pieces' one invokes various kinds of phase change formalism, for example, renormalization theory in cases where a mean field approximation holds (Wallace, 2005), or variants of random network theory where a mean number approximation is applied. More will be said of this below.

Recall that the Shannon uncertainties $H(...)$ are cross-sectional law-of-large-numbers sums of the form $- \sum_k P_k \log[P_k]$, where the P_k constitute a probability distribution. See Cover and Thomas (2006), Ash (1990), or Khinchin (1957) for the standard details, summarized in the Mathematical Appendix.

A formal equivalence class algebra can be constructed by choosing different origin points, a_0, and defining the equivalence of two states, a_m, a_n, by the existence of high probability meaningful paths connecting them to the *same* origin point. Disjoint partition by equivalence class, analogous to orbit equivalence classes for dynamical systems, defines the vertices of the proposed network of cognitive dual languages. Each vertex then represents a different information source dual to a cognitive process. This is not a representation of a neural network as such, or of some circuit in silicon. It is, rather, an abstract set of 'languages' dual to the cognitive biological processes.

This structure generates a groupoid, leading to complicated algebraic properties summarized in the Mathematical Appendix.

A recent series of articles has applied this perspective to cognitive paradigms for gene expression (Wallace and Wallace, 2009, 2010), the regulation of protein folding (Wallace, 2010, 2011a, b), and the production and regulation of the glycan determinants that coat cellular surfaces and, in fact, constitute the principal means of biological information transmission (Wallace, 2012a). Some of these applications will be described in subsequent chapters.

The essential point is that such regulatory machineries can become nodes on a network of interacting information sources whose connections, by crosstalk, become the means for generating shifting, tunable, global broadcasts analogous to neural consciousness that dedicate chosen sets of physiological subsystems to selected problems. We summarize this in the next section.

1.4 The Human Cognome

The human cognome, then, is the overlapping, interpenetrating assembly of cognitive modules within each human and within which each is embedded. The cognome's scale, thus, ranges from the molecular and cellular, through the social and institutional. Here are a few examples, in no particular order.

Immune system
As described, Atlan and Cohen (1998) have proposed an information-theoretic cognitive model of immune function and process, a paradigm incorporating cognitive pattern recognition-and-response behaviors analogous to those of the central nervous system.

From the Atlan/Cohen perspective, the meaning of an antigen can be reduced to the type of response the antigen generates. That is, the meaning of an antigen is functionally defined by the response of the immune system. The meaning of an antigen to the system is discernible in the type of immune response produced, not merely whether or not the antigen is perceived by the receptor repertoire. Because the meaning is defined by the type of response, there is indeed a response repertoire and not only a receptor repertoire.

To account for immune interpretation, Cohen (1992, 2000) has reformulated the cognitive paradigm for the immune system. The immune system can respond to a given antigen in various ways, it has 'options'. Thus, the particular response observed is the outcome of internal processes of weighing and integrating information about the antigen.

In contrast to Burnet's view of the immune response as a simple reflex, it is seen to exercise cognition by the interpolation of a level of information processing between the antigen stimulus and the immune response. A cognitive immune system organizes the information borne by the antigen stimulus within a given context and creates a format suitable for internal processing; the antigen and its context are transcribed internally into the 'chemical language' of the immune system.

The cognitive paradigm suggests a language metaphor to describe immune communication by a string of chemical signals. This metaphor is apt because the human and immune languages can be seen to manifest several similarities such as syntax and abstraction. Syntax, for example, enhances both linguistic and immune meaning.

Although individual words and even letters can have their own meanings, an unconnected subject or an unconnected predicate will tend to mean less than does the sentence generated by their connection.

The immune system creates a 'language' by linking two ontogenetically different classes of molecules in a syntactical fashion. One class of molecules are the T and B cell receptors for antigens. These molecules are not inherited, but are somatically generated in each individual. The other class of molecules responsible for internal information processing is encoded in the individual's germline.

Meaning, i.e., the chosen type of immune response, is the outcome of the concrete connection between the antigen subject and the germline predicate signals.

The transcription of the antigens into processed peptides embedded in a context of germline ancillary signals constitutes the functional language of the immune system. Despite the logic of clonal selection, the immune system does not respond to antigens as they are, but to abstractions of antigens-in-context.

Tumor control

Nunney (1999) has explored cancer occurrence as a function of animal size, suggesting that in larger animals, whose lifespan grows at about the 4/10 power of their cell count, prevention of cancer in rapidly proliferating tissues becomes more difficult in proportion to size. Cancer control requires the development of additional mechanisms and systems to address tumorigenesis as body size increases – a synergistic effect of cell number and organism longevity. Nunney concludes that this pattern may represent a real barrier to the evolution of large, long-lived animals and predicts that those that do evolve have recruited additional controls over those of smaller animals to prevent cancer.

In particular, different tissues may have evolved markedly different tumor control strategies. All of these, however, are likely to be energetically expensive, permeated with different complex signaling strategies, and subject to a multiplicity of reactions to signals, including those related to psychosocial stress. Forlenza and Baum (2000) explore the effects of stress on the full spectrum of tumor control, ranging from DNA damage and control, to apoptosis, immune surveillance, and mutation rate. R. Wallace *et al.*, (2003) argue that this elaborate tumor control strategy, at least in large animals, must be at least as cognitive as the immune system itself, which is one of its components: some comparison must be made with an internal picture of a healthy cell, and a choice made as to response, i.e., none, attempt DNA repair, trigger programmed cell death, engage in full-blown immune attack. This is, from the Atlan/Cohen perspective, the essence of cognition.

The HPA axis

The hypothalamic-pituitary-adrenal (HPA) axis, the flight-or-fight system, is clearly cognitive in the Atlan/Cohen sense. Upon recognition of a new perturbation in the surrounding environment, memory and brain or emotional cognition evaluate and choose from several possible responses: no action needed, flight, fight, helplessness (i.e., flight or fight needed, but not possible). Upon appropriate conditioning, the HPA axis is able to accelerate the decision process, much as the immune system has a more efficient response to second pathogenic challenge once the initial infection has become encoded in immune memory. Certainly hyperreactivity in the context of post-traumatic stress disorder (PTSD) is a well-known example. Chronic

HPA axis activation is deeply implicated in visceral obesity leading to diabetes and heart disease via the leptin/cortisol diurnal cycle (e.g., Bjorntorp, 2001). A more detailed discussion will be given in Chapters 10 and 11.

Blood pressure regulation

Rau and Elbert (2001) review much of the literature on blood pressure regulation, particularly the interaction between baroreceptor activation and central nervous function. The essential point, of course, is that unregulated blood pressure would be quickly fatal in any animal with a circulatory system, a matter as physiologically fundamental as tumor control. Much work over the years has elucidated some of the mechanisms involved: increase in arterial blood pressure stimulates the arterial baroreceptors which in turn elicit the baroreceptor reflex, causing a reduction in cardiac output and in peripheral resistance, returning pressure to its original level. The reflex, however, is not actually this simple: it may be inhibited through peripheral processes, for example, under conditions of high metabolic demand. In addition, higher brain structures modulate this reflex arc, for instance when threat is detected and fight or flight responses are being prepared.

This suggests, then, that blood pressure control cannot be a simple reflex, but is, rather, a broad and actively cognitive modular system which compares a set of incoming signals with an internal reference configuration, and then chooses an appropriate physiological level of blood pressure from a large repertoire of possible levels, i.e., a cognitive process in the Atlan/Cohen sense. The baroreceptors and the baroreceptor reflex are, from this perspective, only one set of a complex array of components making up a larger and more comprehensive cognitive blood pressure regulatory module.

Emotion

Thayer and Lane (2000) summarize the case for what can be described as a cognitive emotional process. Emotions, in their view, are an integrative index of individual adjustment to changing environmental demands, an organismal response to an environmental event that allows rapid mobilization of multiple subsystems. Emotions are the moment-to-moment output of a continuous sequence of behavior, organized around biologically important functions.

Emotions are self-regulatory responses that allow the efficient coordination of the organism for goal-directed behavior. Specific emotions imply specific eliciting stimuli, specific action tendencies, including selective attention to relevant stimuli, and specific reinforcers. When the system works properly, it allows for flexible adaptation of the organism to changing environmental demands, so that an emotional response represents a *selection* of an appropriate response and the inhibition of other less appropriate responses from a more or less broad behavioral repertoire of possible responses. Such choice is the essence of the Atlan and Cohen language metaphor.

Gene expression

Wallace and Wallace (2008, 2009, 2010, 2011) have introduced an explicit cognitive paradigm for gene expression in which an expressed phenotype is seen as a chosen response to inherited epigenetic and impinging environmental signals during development. Epigenetic context affects gene expression and organsimal development by serving as analogs to a tunable catalyst, directing development into different characteristic pathways according to the structure of external signals. The choices necessary at each developmental branch point of the organism (West-Eberhard, 2003, 2005) are, again, the essence of cognition. Considerably more will be said of this in Chapters 4 and 5.

Protein folding regulation

Although amino acid sequence indeed 'predicts' the canonical normal form of a folded protein (e.g., Anfinsen, 1973), the existence of a broad spectrum of protein folding disorders, in the context of 'shock protein' chaperones and related mechanisms, suggests that there is an elaborate cellular cognitive process that recognizes, passes, repairs, and/or eliminates, proteins (Wallace, 2010, 2011a). Chapter 6 will explore these matters in more detail.

The glycome

Following Wallace (2012a), unlike the universal genetic code and ordered protein folding, direct application of Tlusty's rate distortion index theorem method (Tlusty, 2007) to the glycome – the glycan 'kelp bed' that coats the cellular surface and, through interaction with lectin proteins, carries the major share of biological information – produces a *reductio ad absurdum*. From the beginning, a complicated system of chemical cognition is needed so that external information constrains and tunes what would otherwise be a monstrously large 'glycan code error network'. Further, the glycan manufacture machinery itself must be regulated by yet other levels of chemical cognition to ensure that what is produced on the cell surface matches what was actually chosen for production. Finally, the business end of the glycan kelp bed that coats cellular surfaces involves logic gate interactions with lectin proteins that are essential building blocks of cellular cognition. Chapters 7 and 8 will take a more detailed look.

Intrinsically disordered protein logic gates
Intrinsically disordered proteins (IDP) appear far more likely to engage in
functional moonlighting than well-structured proteins. The use of nonrigid
molecule theory to address IDP structure and dynamics produces this result
directly (Wallace, 2011b, 2012b): mirror image subgroup or subgroupoid
tiling matching of the molecular fuzzy lock-and-key can be much richer for
IDPs since the number of possible group or groupoid symmetries can grow
exponentially with molecule length, while tiling matching for 3D structured
proteins is relatively limited. An information catalysis model suggests how
this mechanism can produce a vast spectrum of biological logic gates having subtle properties far beyond familiar AND, OR, XOR, etc. behaviors.
These can be easily stacked to create a broad spectrum of cognitive behaviors. Chapter 9 explores this in more detail.

Sociocultural network
Humans are particularly noted for a hypersociality inevitably enmeshing
them in group processes of decision, i.e., collective cognitive behavior within
a social network, constrained by the embedding context of shared culture.
For humans, culture is truly fundamental. Durham (1991) argues that
genes and culture are two distinct but interacting systems of inheritance
within human populations. Information of both kinds has influence, actual
or potential, over behaviors, creating a real and unambiguous symmetry
between genes and phenotypes, on the one hand, and culture and phenotypes on the other. Genes and culture are best represented as two parallel
lines or tracks of hereditary influence on phenotypes.

Much of hominid evolution can be characterized as an interweaving of
genetic and cultural systems. Genes came to encode for increasing hypersociality, learning, and language skills. The most successful populations
displayed increasingly complex structures that better aided in buffering the
local environment (Bonner, 1980).

Successful human populations seem to have a core of tool usage, sophisticated language, oral tradition, mythology, music, magic, medicine,
and religion, and decision-making skills focused on relatively small fam-
ily/extended family social network groupings. More complex social structures are built on the periphery of this basic object (Richerson and Boyd,
2006). The human species' very identity may rest on its unique evolved
capacities for social mediation and cultural transmission. These are particularly expressed through the cognitive decision-making of small groups
facing changing patterns of threat and opportunity, processes in which we
are all embedded and all participate.

This perspective can easily be expanded to examine large-scale failure in public health using tools similar to those now standard for the study of 'cockpit' malfunction for emergency rooms. See Wallace and Fullilove (2008), and references therein. Chapters 10 and 11 will review some of these matters.

Chapter 2

EXPANDING THE THEORY

2.1 No Free Lunch

Given a set of biological cognitive modules that become linked to solve a
problem – e.g., riding a bicycle in heavy traffic, followed by localized wound
healing – the famous 'no free lunch' theorem of Wolpert and Macready
(1995, 1997) illuminates the next step in the argument. As English (1996)
states the matter:

> ...Wolpert and Macready... have established that there exists no
> generally superior [computational] function optimizer. There is no
> 'free lunch' in the sense that an optimizer 'pays' for superior perfor-
> mance on some functions with inferior performance on others... gains
> and losses balance precisely, and all optimizers have identical average
> performance... [That is] an optimizer has to 'pay' for its superior-
> ity on one subset of functions with inferiority on the complementary
> subset...

Another way of stating this conundrum is to say that a computed solution is simply the product of the information processing of a problem,
and, by a very famous argument, information can never be gained simply
by processing. Thus, a problem, X, is transmitted as a message by an
information processing channel, Y, a computing device, and recoded as an
answer. By the extended argument of the Mathematical Appendix, there
will be a channel coding of Y which, when properly tuned, is *itself* most
efficiently 'transmitted', in a purely formal sense, by the problem – the
'message' X. In general, then, the most efficient coding of the transmission channel, that is, the best algorithm turning a problem into a solution,
will necessarily be highly problem-specific. Thus, there can be no best al-

gorithm for all sets of problems, although there will likely be an optimal algorithm for any given set.

Based on the no free lunch argument, it is clear that different challenges facing an entity must be met by different arrangements of cooperating basic 'low level' cognitive modules. It is possible to make a very abstract picture of this phenomenon, not based on anatomy, but rather on the linkages between the information sources dual to the basic physiological and learned unconscious cognitive modules (UCM). That is, *the remapped network of lower level cognitive modules is reexpressed in terms of the information sources dual to the UCM.* Given two distinct problem classes (e.g., riding a bicycle vs. wound healing), there must be two different 'wirings' of the information sources dual to the available physiological UCM, as in Fig. 2.1, with the network graph edges measured by the amount of information crosstalk between sets of nodes representing the dual information sources. A more formal treatment of such coupling can be given in terms of network information theory (Cover and Thomas, 2006), particularly incorporating the effects of embedding contexts, implied by the 'external' information source Z – signals from the environment.

The possible expansion of a closely linked set of information sources dual to the UCM into a global workspace/broadcast – the occurrence of a kind of 'spandrel' – depends, in this model, on the underlying network topology of the dual information sources and on the strength of the couplings between the individual components of that network.

For random networks the results are well known, based on the work of Erdos and Renyi (1960). Following the review by Spenser (2010) closely (see, e.g., Boccaletti *et al.*, 2006, for more detail), assume there are n network nodes and e edges connecting the nodes, distributed with uniform probability – no nonrandom clustering. Let $G[n, e]$ be the state when there are e edges. The central question is the typical behavior of $G[n, e]$ as e changes from 0 to $(n-2)!/2$. The latter expression is the number of possible pair contacts in a population having n individuals. Another way to say this is to let $G(n, p)$ be the probability space over graphs on n vertices where each pair is adjacent with independent probability p. The behaviors of $G[n, e]$ and $G(n, p)$ where $e = p(n - 2)!/2$ are asymptotically the same.

For 'real world' biological and social structures, one can have $p = f(e, n)$, where f may not be simple or even monotonic. For example, while low e would almost always be associated with low p, beyond some threshold, high e might drive individuals or nodal groups into isolation, decreasing p and producing an 'inverted-U' signal transduction relation akin to stochas-

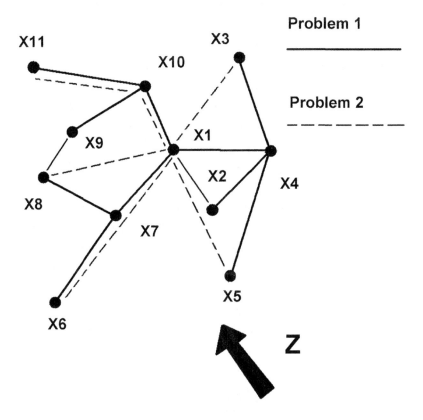

Fig. 2.1   By the no free lunch theorem, two markedly different problems will be optimally solved by two different linkages of available lower level cognitive modules – characterized now by their dual information sources X_j – into different temporary networks of working structures, here represented by crosstalk among those sources rather than by the physiological UCM themselves. The embedding information source Z represents the influence of external signals whose effects can be, at least formally, accounted for by network information theory.

tic resonance. Something like this would account for Fechner's law stating that perception of sensory signals often scales as the log of the signal intensity.

For the simple random case, however, we can parameterize as $p = c/n$. The graph with $n/2$ edges then corresponds to $c = 1$. The essential finding is that the behavior of the random network has three sections:

1. If $c < 1$, all the linked subnetworks are very small, *and no global broadcast can take place*.

2. If $c = 1$, there is a single large interlinked component of a size $\approx n^{2/3}$.

3. If $c > 1$, then there is a single large component of size yn – a global broadcast – where y is the positive solution to the equation

$$\exp(-cy) = 1 - y. \tag{2.1}$$

Then

$$y = \frac{W(-c/\exp(c)) + c}{c}, \tag{2.2}$$

where W is the Lambert W function.

The solid line in Fig. 2.2 shows y as a function of c, representing the fraction of network nodes that are incorporated into the interlinked giant component – a de facto global broadcast for interacting UCM. To the left of $c = 1$ there is no giant component, and large scale cognitive process is not possible.

The dotted line, however, represents the fraction of nodes in the giant component for a highly nonrandom network, a star-of-stars-of-stars (SoS) in which every node is directly or indirectly connected with every other one. For such a topology there is no threshold, only a single giant component, showing that the emergence of a giant component in a network of information sources dual to the UCM is dependent on a network topology that may itself be tunable. We will obtain a generalization of this result by means of an index theorem argument below.

2.2 Multiple Broadcasts, Punctuated Detection

The random network development above is predicated on there being a variable average number of fixed-strength linkages between components. Clearly, the mutual information measure of crosstalk is not inherently fixed, but can continuously vary in magnitude. This suggests a a parameterized renormalization. In essence, the modular network structure linked by mutual information interactions has a topology depending on the degree of interaction of interest.

Define an interaction parameter ω, a real positive number, and look at geometric structures defined in terms of linkages set to zero if mutual information is less than, and 'renormalized' to unity if greater than, ω. Any given ω will define a regime of giant components of network elements linked by mutual information greater than or equal to it.

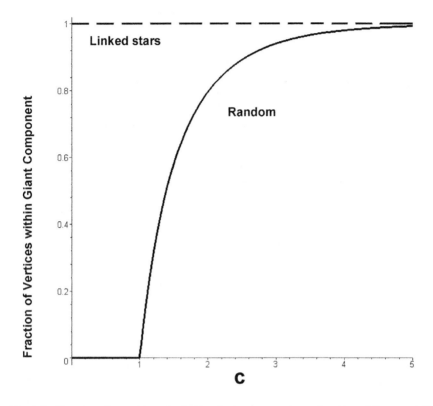

Fig. 2.2 Fraction of network nodes in the giant component as a function of the crosstalk coupling parameter c. The solid line represents a random graph, the dotted line a star-of-stars-of-stars network in which all nodes are interconnected, showing that the dynamics of giant component emergence are highly dependent on an underlying network topology that, for UCM, may itself be tunable. For the random graph, a strength of $c < 1$ precludes emergence of a larger-scale 'global' broadcast.

Now invert the argument: A given topology for the giant component will, in turn, define some critical value, ω_C, so that network elements interacting by mutual information less than that value will be unable to participate, i.e., will be locked out and not be 'consciously' perceived. Thus ω is a tunable, syntactically-dependent, detection limit that depends critically on the instantaneous topology of the giant component of linked cognitive modules defining the global broadcast. That topology is, fundamentally, the basic tunable syntactic filter across the underlying modular structure, and variation in ω is only one aspect of a much more general topological shift. Further analysis can be given in terms of a topological rate distortion manifold (Wallace and Fullilove, 2008; Glazebrook and Wallace, 2009a, b).

There is considerable empirical evidence from fMRI brain imaging and many other experiments to show that individual animal consciousness – restricted by necessity of a time constant near 100 ms. – involves a single, shifting and tunable, global broadcast, a matter leading to the phenomenon of inattentional blindness. Multiple cognitive submodules within systems not constrained to the 100 ms time range, for example, institutions – individuals, departments, formal and informal workgroups – by contrast, can do more than one thing, and indeed, are usually required to multitask. Clearly, then, multiple workspace global broadcasts lessen the probability of inattentional blindness, if there is time to support them, but do not eliminate it, and introduce critical failure modes related to the degradation of information transmitted between global broadcasts.

It is necessary to postulate a set of crosstalk information measures between cognitive submodules, each associated with its own tunable giant component having its own special topology.

Again, although animal consciousness, with its 100 ms. time constant, seems restricted to a single tunable global broadcast, it is clear that slower physiological global broadcast analogs would permit individual subsystems, or localized sets of such subsystems, to engage in more than one global broadcast at a time, to multitask, in the same sense that workgroups within an institution will usually be given more than one task at a time. Thus, the immune system can be expected to simultaneously engage in wound healing, attack invading microorganisms, and conduct neuroimmuno dialog and routine tissue maintenance tasks (Cohen, 2000).

Following, again, the arguments of Wallace and Fullilove (2008), the argument can be expanded.

Suppose, now, a set of giant components of interacting cognitive physiological submodules at some time, k, is characterized by a set of parameters $\Omega_k \equiv (\omega_1^k, ..., \omega_m^k)$. Fixed parameter values define a particular giant component set having a particular set of topological structures. Suppose that, over a sequence of times, the set of giant components can be characterized by a possibly coarse-grained path $x_n = (\Omega_0, \Omega_1, ..., \Omega_{n-1})$ having significant serial correlations permitting definition of an adiabatically, piecewise stationary, ergodic (APSE) information source X.

Suppose a set of (external or internal) signals impinging on the set of giant components is also highly structured and forms another APSE information source Y. Then it becomes possible to define joint and conditional Shannon uncertainties leading to an iterated chain rule argument, complicated by the necessity of information transfer between the multiple, shifting spotlights characterizing the interacting giant components. To reiterate, a major possible source of pathology would be distortion in the transmission of information between interacting global broadcasts.

2.3 Metabolic Constraints

The information sources dual to unconscious cognitive modules represented in Fig. 2.1 are not independent, but are correlated, so that a joint information source can be defined having the properties

$$H(X_1, ..., X_n) \leq \sum_{j=1}^{n} H(X_j). \tag{2.3}$$

This result is known as the information chain rule (e.g., Cover and Thomas, 2006), and has profound implications: Feynman (2000) describes in great detail how information and free energy have an inherent duality. Feynman, in fact, defines information precisely as the free energy needed to erase a message. The argument is surprisingly direct (e.g., Bennett, 1988), and for very simple systems it is easy to design a small (idealized) machine that turns the information within a message directly into usable work – free energy. Information is a form of free energy and the construction and transmission of information within living things consumes metabolic free energy, with inevitable – usually considerable – losses via the second law of thermodynamics. This latter point will prove to be central.

Information catalysis arises most simply via the information theory chain rule. Restricting the argument to two information sources, X and Y, one can define jointly typical paths $z_i = (x_i, y_i)$ having the joint information source uncertainty $H(X, Y)$ satisfying $H(X, Y) = H(X) + H(Y|X) \leq H(X) + H(Y)$. Of necessity, then,

$$H(X, Y) \leq H(X) + H(Y) \, if \, H(Y) \neq 0.$$

Within a biological structure, however, there will be an ensemble of possible reactions, driven by the intensity of available metabolic free energy, M, so that, taking $\hat{H}$ as representing an average,

$$\hat{H}(X, Y) < \hat{H}(X) + \hat{H}(Y). \tag{2.4}$$

This is a very general result that, by the homology between information and free energy, leads to a model in which interacting biological signals can 'canalize' the overall behavior of the system: Interaction consumes less metabolic free energy than signal isolation.

Let $Q(\kappa M) \geq 0, Q(0) = 0$ represent a monotonic increasing function of the intensity measure of available metabolic free energy M, and C be the maximum channel capacity available to the cognitive biological processes of interest. One would expect

$$\hat{H} = \frac{\int_0^C H \exp[-H/Q]dH}{\int_0^C \exp[-H/Q]dH} = \frac{Q[\exp(C/Q) - 1] - C}{\exp(C/Q) - 1}. \qquad (2.5)$$

κ is an inverse energy intensity scaling constant that may be quite small indeed, a consequence of the typically massive entropic translation losses between the metabolic free energy consumed by the physical processes that instantiate information and any actual measure of that information.

Near $M = 0$, expand Q as a Taylor series, with a first term $Q \approx \kappa M$.

This expression tops out quite rapidly with increases in either C or Q, producing energy- and channel capacity-limited results

$$\hat{H} = Q(\kappa M), C/2. \qquad (2.6)$$

Then, expanding Q near zero, the two limiting relations imply

$$Q(\kappa M_{X,Y}) < Q(\kappa M_X) + Q(\kappa M_Y) \rightarrow M_{X,Y} < M_X + M_Y \,,$$

$$C_{X,Y} < C_X + C_Y \,. \qquad (2.7)$$

The channel capacity constraint can be parsed further for a noisy Gaussian channel. Then (Cover and Thomas, 2006)

$$C = 1/2 \log[1 + \mathcal{P}/\sigma^2] \approx 1/2 \mathcal{P}/\sigma^2 \qquad (2.8)$$

for small $\mathcal{P}/\sigma^2$, where $\mathcal{P}$ is the 'power constraint' such that $E(X^2) < \mathcal{P}$ and σ^2 is the noise variance. Assuming information sources X and Y act on the same scale, so that noise variances are the same and quite large, then, taking $\mathcal{P} = Q(\kappa M)$, since channel power is determined by available metabolic free energy, and

$$Q(\kappa M_{X,Y}) < Q(\kappa M_X) + Q(\kappa M_Y).$$

Both limiting inequalities are, then, free energy relations leading to a kind of 'reaction canalization' in which a set of lower level cognitive modules consumes less metabolic free energy if information crosstalk among them is permitted than under conditions of individual signal isolation.

The global broadcast mechanisms of consciousness and its slower physiological generalizations make an arch of this spandrel, using the lowered metabolic free energy requirement of crosstalk interaction between low level cognitive modules as the springboard for launching (sometimes) rapid, tunable, more highly correlated, multiple global broadcasts that link those modules to solve problems.

2.4   Environmental Signals

Lower level cognitive modules operate within larger, highly structured, environmental signals and other constraints whose regularities may also have a recognizable grammar and syntax, represented in Fig. 2.1 by an embedding information source Z. Under such a circumstance the splitting criterion for three jointly typical sequences is given by the classic relation of network information theory (Cover and Thomas, 2006, Theorem 15.2.3)

$$I(X_1, X_2|Z) = H(Z) + H(X_1|Z) + H(X_2|Z) - H(X_1, X_2, Z) \qquad (2.9)$$

that generalizes as

$$I(X_1, ..., X_n|Z) = H(Z) + \sum_{j=1}^{n} H(X_j|Z) - H(X_1, ..., X_n, Z). \qquad (2.10)$$

More complicated multivariate typical sequences are treated much the same (e.g., El Gamal and Kim, 2010). Given a basic set of interacting information sources $(X_1, ..., X_k)$ that one partitions into two ordered sets $X(\mathcal{J})$ and $X(\mathcal{J}')$, then the splitting criterion becomes $H[X(\mathcal{J}|\mathcal{J}')]$. Extension to a greater number of ordered sets is straightforward.

Then the joint splitting criterion – I, H above – however it may be expressed as a composite of the underlying information sources and their interactions, satisfies a relation like the first expression in Eq. (1.2), where $N(n)$ is the number of high probability jointly typical paths of length n, and the theory carries through, now incorporating the effects of external signals as the information source Z.

Chapter 3

DYNAMIC 'REGRESSION' MODELS

3.1 The Simplest Approach

Given the splitting criteria $I(X_1, ..., X_n|Z)$ or $H[X(\mathcal{J}|\mathcal{J}')]$ as above, the essential point is that these are the limit, for large n, of the expression $\log[N(n)]/n$, where $N(n)$ is the number of jointly typical paths of the interacting information sources of length n. Again, as Feynman (2000) argues at great length, information is simply another form of free energy, and its dynamics can be expressed using a formalism similar to Onsager's nonequilibrium thermodynamics. This is particularly apt in view of the enormous levels of free energy needed to physically instantiate information transmission. The argument is direct.

First, the physical model. Let $F(K)$ be the free energy density of a physical system, K the normalized temperature, V the volume and $Z(K, V)$ the *partition function* defined from the Hamiltonian characterizing energy states E_i. Then

$$Z(V, K) \equiv \sum_i \exp[-E_i(V)/K], \tag{3.1}$$

and

$$F(K) = \lim_{V \to \infty} -K \frac{\log[Z(V, K))}{V} \equiv \frac{\log[\hat{Z}(K, V)]}{V}.$$

If a nonequilibrium physical system is parameterized by a set of variables $\{K_i\}$, then the *empirical Onsager equations* are defined in terms of the gradient of the entropy S as

$$dK_j/dt = \sum_i L_{i,j} \partial S/\partial K_i, \tag{3.2}$$

where the $L_{i,j}$ are empirical constants. For a physical system having microreversibility, $L_{i,j} = L_{j,i}$. For an information source where, for example, in English the three-character string 'the' has a much different probability than does the string 'eht', no such microreversibility is possible, and no 'reciprocity relations' can apply.

For stochastic systems this generalizes to the set of stochastic differential equations

$$dK_t^j = \sum_i [L_{j,i}(t, ...\partial S/\partial K^i...)dt + \sigma_{j,i}(t, ...\partial S/\partial K^i)dB_t^i] =$$

$$L(t, K^1, ..., K^n)dt + \sum_i \sigma(t, K^1, ..., K^n)dB_t^i, \quad (3.3)$$

where terms have been collected and expressed in terms of the driving parameters. The dB_t^i represent different kinds of 'noise' whose characteristics are usually expressed by their quadratic variation. See any standard text for definitions, examples, and details. A summary is provided in the Mathematical Appendix.

The essential trick is to recognize that, for the splitting criteria $I(X_1, ..., X_n|Z)$ or $H[X(\mathcal{J}|\mathcal{J}')]$, the role of information as a form of free energy, and the corresponding limit in $\log[N(n)]/n$, make it possible to define entropy-analogs as the Legendre transforms (Landau and Lifshitz, 2007; Pettini, 2007)

$$S \equiv I(...K^i...) - \sum_j K^j \partial I/\partial K^j,$$

$$S \equiv H[X(\mathcal{J}|\mathcal{J}')] - \sum_j K^j \partial H[X(\mathcal{J}|\mathcal{J}')]/\partial K^j,$$

$$S \propto M_{\mathcal{J}|\mathcal{J}'} - \sum_j K^j \partial M_{\mathcal{J}|\mathcal{J}'}/\partial K^j, \quad (3.4)$$

where the last relation invokes the embedding metabolic free energies that instantiate the actual mechanisms by which information is transmitted.

The basic dynamic 'regression equations' for the system of Figs. 2.1 and 2.2, driven by a set of external 'sensory' and other, internal, signal parameters $\mathbf{K} = (K^1, ..., K^n)$ that may be measured by the information source uncertainty of other information sources, is then precisely the set of Eqs. (3.3) above.

In essence, the fundamental picture becomes reversed, and the actual driving metabolic free energy measures M_X are now seen as indexed by the source uncertainties $H[X]$. The different M_X become each other's embedding environments in an analog to coevolutionary dynamics.

Several features emerge directly from invoking such a coevolutionary approach. The first involves Pettini's (2007) topological hypothesis: A fundamental change in the underlying topology of a system characterized by any free energy-like 'Morse function' is a necessary condition for the kind of phase transition shown in Fig. 2.2. What seems clear from the neurological context is that a converse topological tuning of the threshold for the global broadcast phase transition is possible.

Second, there are several obvious possible dynamic patterns:

1. Setting Eq. (3.3) equal to zero and solving for stationary points gives attractor states since the noise terms preclude unstable equilibria.

2. This system may converge to limit cycle or pseudorandom 'strange attractor' behaviors in which the system seems to chase its tail endlessly within a limited venue – a kind of 'Red Queen' pathology.

3. What is converged to in both cases is not a simple state or limit cycle of states. Rather, it is an equivalence class, or set of them, of highly dynamic information sources coupled by mutual interaction through crosstalk. Thus 'stability' in this structure represents particular patterns of ongoing dynamics rather than some identifiable static configuration.

We are deeply enmeshed in highly recursive phenomenological stochastic differential equations (as in, e.g., Zhu *et al.*, 2007), but in a dynamic rather than static manner. The objects of this dynamical system are equivalence classes of information sources, rather than simple 'stationary states' of a dynamical or reactive chemical system. The necessary conditions of the asymptotic limit theorems of communication theory have beaten the mathematical thicket back one layer.

Third, as Champagnat *et al.* (2006) note, shifts between the quasi-equilibria of a coevolutionary system can be addressed by the large deviations formalism. See the Mathematical Appendix for an introduction to the topic. The issue of dynamics drifting away from trajectories predicted by the canonical equation can be investigated by considering the asymptotic of the probability of 'rare events' for the sample paths of the diffusion.

'Rare events' are the diffusion paths drifting far away from the direct solutions of the canonical equation. The probability of such rare events is governed by a large deviation principle: when a critical parameter (designated ϵ) goes to zero, the probability that the sample path of the diffusion is close to a given rare path ϕ decreases exponentially to 0 with rate $\mathcal{I}(\phi)$, where the 'rate function' $\mathcal{I}$ can be expressed in terms of the parameters of the diffusion.

This result can be used to study long-time behavior of the diffusion process when there are multiple attractive singularities. Under proper conditions the most likely path followed by the diffusion when exiting a basin of attraction is the one minimizing the rate function $\mathcal{I}$ over all the appropriate trajectories. The time needed to exit the basin is of the order $\exp(\mathcal{V}/\epsilon)$ where $\mathcal{V}$ is a quasi-potential representing the minimum of the rate function $\mathcal{I}$ over all possible trajectories.

An essential fact of large deviations theory is that the rate function $\mathcal{I}$ which Champagnat *et al.* invoke can almost always be expressed as a kind of entropy, that is, having the canonical form

$$\mathcal{I} = -\sum_j P_j \log(P_j) \qquad (3.5)$$

for some probability distribution. This result goes under a number of names; Sanov's theorem, Cramer's theorem, the Gartner–Ellis theorem, the Shannon–McMillan theorem, and so forth (Dembo and Zeitouni, 1998).

These arguments are very much in the direction of Eq. (3.3), now seen as subject to internally-driven large deviations *that can themselves be described as information sources*, providing $K = f(\mathcal{I})$-parameters that can trigger punctuated shifts between quasi-stable modes. Thus both external signals, characterized by the information source Z, and internal 'ruminations', characterized by an information source $\mathcal{I}$, can provide K-parameters that serve to drive the system to different quasi-equilibrium 'conscious attention states' in a highly punctuated manner, if they are of sufficient magnitude to overcome the topological renormalization ω-constraints described in Section 2.2.

A schematic of these ideas has become common currency in systems biology, and Fig. 3.1, adapted from Fig. 1 of the famous paper by Kitano (2004), provides a somewhat mechanistic picture, including several possible modes. Taking a two-dimensional parameterization, so that there are two K_j, different basins of attraction in parameter space show system response to perturbation: (A) Return to a periodic (or chaotic) attractor. (B) Transition to a new attractor. (C) Stochastic process or external information source $\mathcal{I}$ influences the trajectory. (D) Return to a point attractor. (E) An unstable random walk to another basin of attraction. This should be compared with Fig. 2.1 that represents two of the different network topologies of the dual information sources behind the parameterization.

Figure 3.1 then presents, in parameter space, several of the different 'no free lunch' arrangements of unconscious cognitive modules, as in Fig. 2.1, that unite to address problems facing the organism.

More generally, however, following the deep topological arguments of Section 2.2, setting Eq. (3.3) to zero generates an *index theorem* (Hazewinkel, 2002) in the sense of Atiyah and Singer (1963). Such an object

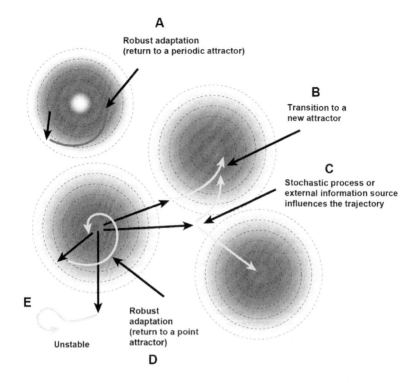

Fig. 3.1 Adapted from Kitano (2004). Using a two-dimensional schematic, different basins of attraction in parameter space show system response to perturbation. A. Return to a periodic (or chaotic) attractor. B. Transition to a new attractor. C. Stochastic process or external information source $\mathcal{I}$ influences the trajectory. D. Return to a point attractor. E. Unstable random walk to another basin of attraction. Compare with Fig. 2.1 which represents the different network topologies of the dual information sources that are behind the parameterization.

relates analytic results – the solutions to the equations – to an underlying set of topological structures that are eigenmodes of a complicated Ω-network geometric operator whose spectrum represents the possible multiple global broadcast states of the system. This structure, and its dynamics, do not really have simple mechanical or electrical system analogs.

Index theorems, in this context, instantiate relations between 'conserved' quantities – here, the quasi-equilibria of basins of attraction in parameter space – and underlying topological form – here, the cognitive network conformations of Fig. 2.1. Section 1.3, however, described how

that network was itself defined in terms of equivalence classes of meaningful paths that, in turn, defined groupoids, a significant generalization of the
group symmetries more familiar to physicists.

The approach, then, in a sense – via the groupoid construction – generalizes the famous relation between group symmetries and conservation laws
uncovered by E. Noether that has become the central foundation of modern physics (Byers, 1999). Thus, this work proposes a kind of Noetherian
(NER-terian) statistical dynamics of the living state. The saving grace of
the method, perhaps, is that it represents the fitting of dynamic regression-
like statistical models based on the asymptotic limit theorems of information theory to data, and does not presume to be a 'real' picture of the
underlying systems and their time behaviors: biology is not relativity theory.

As with simple fitted regression equations, actual scientific inference
is done most often by comparing the same systems under different conditions, and different systems under the same conditions: statistics is not
science, and one can easily imagine the necessity of 'nonparametric' or
'non-Noetherian' models.

Finally, an essential perspective of the Baars global workspace/global
broadcast model of animal consciousness is the role of contexts in defining
the 'riverbanks' confining the stream of individual consciousness. The most
essential context for the dynamic global broadcasts associated with human
pathophysiology is the embedding cultural milieu that most distinguishes
humans from other animals. Richerson and Boyd (2006), for example, argue persuasively that culture is as much a part of human biology as the
enamel on our teeth and bipedal locomotion. That is, culture and human
biology are inextricably linked. Pathophysiology involves developmental
trajectories driven by cognitive processes of gene expression (e.g., Wallace
and Wallace, 2010) that, in the sense of Fig. 2.1, respond to environmental
signals largely defined by cultural context as mitigated by social interaction and the power relations between groups. Expressing the regularities of
sociocultural interaction in terms of the grammar and syntax of an information source would permit their incorporation into the dynamics of Eq.
(3.3) in a natural manner. Clearly, then, the 'riverbank' nature of cultural
pattern and power relations that directs the stream of human pathophysiology arises from the difference in time scales between normal physiological
process and the rate of change of culture, catastrophic events aside.

3.2   A Rate Distortion Reformulation

Real-time dynamics

Real-time biological problems are inherently rate distortion problems, and it becomes possible to reformulate the underlying theory from that perspective. The implementation of a complex cognitive structure, say a sequence of control orders generated by some regulatory dual information source Y, having output $y^n = y_1, y_2, ...$ is 'digitized' in terms of the observed behavior of the regulated system, say the sequence $b^n = b_1, b_2, ...$ The b_i are thus what happens in real time, the actual impact of the cognitive structure on its embedding environment. Assume each b^n is then deterministically retranslated back into a reproduction of the original control signal, $b^n \to \hat{y}^n = \hat{y}_1, \hat{y}_2, ...$

Define a distortion measure $d(y, \hat{y})$ that compares the original to the retranslated path. See the Mathematical Appendix for examples. Suppose that with each path y^n and b^n-path retranslation into the y-language, denoted $\hat{y}^n$, there are associated individual, joint, and conditional probability distributions $p(y^n), p(\hat{y}^n), p(y^n|\hat{y}^n)$.

The average distortion is defined as

$$D \equiv \sum_{y^n} p(y^n) d(y^n, \hat{y}^n) . \tag{3.6}$$

It is possible, using the distributions given above, to define the information transmitted from the incoming Y to the outgoing $\hat{Y}$ process using the Shannon source uncertainty of the strings:

$$I(Y, \hat{Y}) \equiv H(Y) - H(Y|\hat{Y}) = H(Y) + H(\hat{Y}) - H(Y, \hat{Y}).$$

If there is no uncertainty in Y, given the retranslation $\hat{Y}$, then no information is lost, and the regulated system is perfectly under control. In general, this will not be true.

The *information rate distortion function* $R(D)$ for a source Y with a distortion measure $d(y, \hat{y})$ is defined as

$$R(D) = \min_{p(y,\hat{y}); \sum_{(y,\hat{y})} p(y)p(y|\hat{y})d(y,\hat{y}) \leq D} I(Y, \hat{Y}) . \tag{3.7}$$

The Mathematical Appendix provides more detail.

The minimization is over all conditional distributions $p(y|\hat{y})$ for which the joint distribution $p(y, \hat{y}) = p(y)p(y|\hat{y})$ satisfies the average distortion constraint (i.e., average distortion $\leq D$).

The *rate distortion theorem* states that $R(D)$ *is the minimum necessary rate of information transmission – essentially channel capacity – which ensures the transmission does not exceed average distortion* D (Cover and

Thomas, 2006). The rate distortion function has been calculated for a number of systems. Cover and Thomas (2006) show that $R(D)$ is necessarily a decreasing convex function of D, that is, always a reverse J-shaped curve. This is a critical observation, since convexity is an exceptionally powerful mathematical condition (Ellis, 1985; Rockafellar, 1970).

Recall, now, the relation between information source uncertainty and channel capacity. First,

$$H[\mathbf{X}] \leq C, \tag{3.8}$$

where H is the uncertainty of the source X and C the channel capacity. Recall that C is defined according to the relation

$$C \equiv \max_{P(X)} I(X|Y), \tag{3.9}$$

where $P(X)$ is the probability distribution of the message chosen so as to maximize the rate of information transmission along a channel Y.

The rate distortion function places limits on information source uncertainty. Thus distortion measures can drive information system dynamics. That is, the rate distortion function itself has a homological relation to free energy density. This allows a 'more natural' reformulation of the coevolutionary arguments.

The motivation for this approach is the observation that a Gaussian channel with noise variance σ^2 and zero mean has a rate distortion function $R(D) = 1/2 \log[\sigma^2/D]$ using the squared distortion measure. Defining a 'rate distortion entropy' as the Legendre transform

$$S_R = R(D) - DdR(D)/dD = 1/2 \log[\sigma^2/D] + 1/2,$$

the simplest nonequilibrium Onsager equation is

$$dD/dt = -\mu dS_R/dD = \mu/2D,$$

where t is the time and μ is a diffusion coefficient. By inspection,

$$D(t) = \sqrt{\mu t},$$

which is very precisely the solution to the diffusion equation.

Some thought shows this to be an exceedingly fundamental result. It is driven by the convex nature of the rate distortion function, so that similar outcomes – D growing monotonically with time in the absence of energy input – will always occur, and provides an important justification for the next iterations of the argument, in which energy input is allowed, and equilibrium is possible. Most simply, take the nonequilibrium Onsager equation for a Gaussian channel as

$$dD/dt = -\mu dS_R/dD - F, F > 0,$$

where F represents a monotonic increasing function of input free energy intensity. At equilibrium, when $dD/dt = 0$,

$$D_{equilib} = \frac{\mu}{2F}.$$

The equilibrium value of the average distortion is inversely proportional to the index of rate of metabolic free energy availability, suggesting that the aerobic transition may have enabled evolution of increasingly elaborate and effective molecular, cellular, and higher order regulatory systems.

For radar systems, it is well known that F is proportional to the square root of the beam energy.

Rate distortion coevolution

The coevolution model above can be conceptually simplified in terms the rate distortion functions for mutual crosstalk between different cognitive submodules, the effect of contact with the embedding environment, and the effect of the organism on that environment, using the homology of the rate distortion function itself with free energy.

Given different cognitive subprocesses, 1...s, within or embedding the organism, the quantities of special interest thus become the mutual rate distortion functions $R_{i,j}$ characterizing communication (and the average distortions $D_{i,j}$) between them, and $R(D)$, representing the distortion between cognitive intent and actual impact of the entire system. The essential parameters remain the characteristic time constants of each process, $\tau_j, j = 1...s$, and the overall, embedding, 'communication free energy density' representing the maximum possible information available to the multicomponent system from the embedding environment. The distortion between overall organism impact and intent is, in this formulation, taken as simply an additional parameter.

Taking the Q^β to run over all the relevant parameters and mutual rate distortion functions (including distortion measures $D_{i,j}$ and D), the expression for 'entropy' is the Legendre transform

$$S_R^\beta \equiv R_\beta - \sum_\alpha Q^\alpha \partial R_\beta / \partial Q^\alpha \,, \tag{3.10}$$

generalizing Eq. (3.4).

Equation (3.3) accordingly becomes

$$dQ_t^\alpha = \sum_\beta [L_\beta(t, ...\partial S_R^\beta / \partial Q^\alpha ...)dt + \sigma_\beta(t, ...\partial S_R^\beta / \partial Q^\alpha ...)dB_t^\beta] \,, \tag{3.11}$$

where, again, β ranges over the indices of the $R_{i,j}$ and $R(D)$.

Here, the equation explicitly models the roles of crosstalk within the organism, the effect of the organism on the environment, the inherent time constants of the different cognitive modules, and the overall information available from the embedding environment, now taken as a kind of metabolic free energy measure.

This is a very complicated structure indeed, but the general dynamical behaviors will obviously be analogous to those described earlier. For example, setting Eq. (3.11) to zero gives the 'coevolutionary stable states' of a system of interacting cognitive modules in terms of channel capacity, average distortions, system time constants, and measures of free energy density characterizing information available from the environment. Again, limit cycles and strange attractors seem possible as well. What is converged to is a dynamic behavior pattern, not some fixed 'state'. Such a system will display highly punctuated dynamics almost exactly akin to resilience domain shifts in ecosystems, as described by Eq. (3.5).

3.3　Multiple Time Scales

Cognitive biological systems can face numerous 'real' times. Think of a student riding a bicycle in heavy traffic: proper strategies – generalized languages – across multiple timescales are critical, including those of (1) the immediate traffic pattern, (2) the study time needed for passing exams, (3) the time necessary for advancement in a chosen profession, and so on.

Some clues as to the likely subtleties can be found through an elementary calculation.

Let $R(D)$ the rate distortion function describing the relation between cognitive system intent and actual impact, essentially a channel capacity and information transmission rate between the organism or subsystem and the structures it is attempting to affect, and let τ be the characteristic 'real time' of the overall system. Let $\mathcal{H}$ be the total rate of available information telling the cognitive structure what is happening in real time. $\tau R(D)$ and $\tau \mathcal{H}$ are thus basic energy measures. The fundamental assumption is that the probability density function associated with a particular value of $\tau R(D)$ will be given by the classic relation

$$Pr[\tau R(D), \tau \mathcal{H}] = \frac{\exp[-R(D)\tau/\kappa\mathcal{H}\tau]}{\int_0^\infty \exp[-R(D)\tau/\kappa\mathcal{H}\tau]dR}, \qquad (3.12)$$

where κ might represent something like an efficiency measure of information usage. The 'real time' measure τ divides out in this formulation.

Then

$$< R >= \int_0^\infty R Pr[R, \mathcal{H}] dR = \kappa \mathcal{H} .$$ (3.13)

By the arguments above, limits on incoming information $\mathcal{H}$ resulting in limits on $< R >$ will express themselves in limits on the richness of system behavior.

In the case that R and $\mathcal{H}$ have different characteristic times, say τ_R and $\tau_\mathcal{H}$, then κ in the above equations is replaced by

$$\hat{\kappa} = \kappa \frac{\tau_\mathcal{H}}{\tau_R} .$$ (3.14)

Thus the existence of different characteristic timescales for cognitive response and for the pattern of incoming information on which the cognitive structure must act can significantly complicate behavioral dynamics. In particular, decline in the characteristic time of incoming information relative to the characteristic response time of the cognitive system can express itself in punctuated decline in the spectrum of possible cognitive behaviors, as described in the next section.

3.4   Incoming Information

The denominator of Eq. (3.12) itself has the form of a partition function leading to a free energy measure:

$$\mathcal{Z} \equiv \int_0^\infty \exp[-R/\kappa\mathcal{H}] dR ,$$ (3.15)

defining a kind of free energy as

$$\mathcal{F} \equiv -\kappa\mathcal{H} \log[\mathcal{Z}] .$$ (3.16)

Changes in $\kappa\mathcal{H}$, in analogy to phase transition in physical systems, can then trigger punctuated changes in the overall ability of the system to match intent to performance, following Landau's ideas (Landau and Lifshitz, 2007; Pettini, 2007).

The essence of Landau's insight was that phase transitions without latent heat – second order transitions – were usually in the context of a significant symmetry change in the physical states of a system, with one phase, at higher temperature, being far more symmetric than the other. A symmetry is lost in the transition, a phenomenon called spontaneous symmetry breaking. The greatest possible set of symmetries in a physical system is that of the Hamiltonian describing its energy states. Usually, states accessible at lower temperatures will lack symmetries available at higher temperatures, so that the lower temperature phase is the less symmetric: the randomization of higher temperatures ensures that higher symmetry/energy states will then be accessible to the system.

At the lower temperature an order parameter must be introduced to describe the system's physical states – some extensive quantity like magnetization. The order parameter will vanish at higher temperatures, involving more symmetric states, and will be different from zero in the less symmetric lower temperature phase.

A more systematic analysis of Landau's approach will be given in Chapter 6. The essential point here is that declines in the quality of incoming information – $\mathcal{H}$ – can 'freeze' a complicated cognitive system into a kind of (possibly pathological) ground state, in a highly punctuated manner.

The general argument can clearly be applied as well to information exchanges between cognitive modules within an organism.

It is important to realize that this 'ground state' phase transition is as fundamental an information theory necessary condition constraint as are the ubiquity of noise and crosstalk. We will return to it in Chapter 10, in the context of the evolutionary adaptations needed to address it, or which have been exapted from it as another arch built from a spandrel. The particular concern of Chapter 10 is the hypothalamic-pituitary-adrenal (HPA) axis that programs flight or fight responses, but many other physiological mechanisms probably follow from, or use, ground state phase transitions.

3.5   Pathologies

For interacting, highly parallel, real time cognitive biological systems or subsystems, one measure of deterioration in the communication with the embedding environment – which may include other parts of the organism itself – is the decline of a rate distortion function $R(D)$ consequent on increase of the average distortion D between (sub)system intent and actual (sub)system impact. In the context of some fixed expected response time τ, this acts to lower an *internal* 'cognitive temperature'. The cognitive process, from the arguments of Section 3.4, is then driven to simpler and less-rich behaviors, and ultimately condenses to some dysfunctional 'absolute zero' configuration, possibly in a highly punctuated manner. Lowering the quality of incoming information leads to greater distortion and, given the real time constraint, this lowers $R(D)$ and drives the internal state of the system to its ground configuration.

A slightly different picture emerges by considering the amount of information coming from an embedding environment – or other parts of the organism itself – per unit time as fixed, and expect the cognitive process(es) to respond to that information with a minimum of distortion in the difference between its (their) intent and the actual effect. Then the *response time* becomes lengthened, possibly in a highly punctuated manner. This is equivalent to setting $\tau_R = 1$ in Eq. (3.14) and allowing $\tau_\mathcal{H}$ to increase until $< R >$ is sufficiently large. Long response times, however, may not be tolerable in a highly stressed organism.

These results characterize a relatively simple class of failure modes, particularly for systems or subsystems composed of very many interacting cognitive subcomponents. Taking an ontological perspective, the possibility of much more subtle failures – forms of developmental disorders – becomes evident.

Some further insight into possible pathologies can be gained by reconsidering Eq. (3.11) in terms of the distortion measures $D, D_{i,j}$. Solving for equilibrium conditions, it is important to recognize that D, the distortion between system intent and system performance, is to be minimized under the constraints that $D_{i,j} \leq D_{i,j}^{max} \, \forall \, i, j$, given the constraint equation defined by setting $dD/dt = 0$. If some $D_{i,j}$ exceeds its allowable maximum, the system can collapse: think excessive blood pressure in response to stress. This is a complicated problem in Kuhn–Tucker optimization that generalizes the Lagrange multiplier method under inequality (e.g., Nocedal and Wright, 1999). The essential point is that there may be no solution to the optimization problem that allows all $D_{i,j}$ to remain below allowable limits. We will return to this point in a discussion of treatment side effects in Chapter 10.

Cognitive biological structures necessarily undergo developmental trajectories, from an initial configuration to a final 'phenotype' that is either some fixed 'answer' or else a desired dynamic behavior. These are affected, not only by the desires of the genetic (or epigenetic) 'programmer' or the underlying limitations of the system, but also by the distortion between intent and impact, by the degree of information actually available from the environment, and by the effects of epigenetic 'noxious exposures' that may not be random, resulting in pathological phenotypes. How are these pathologies to be redressed? The general argument of Eq. (3.5) that applies here as well can be directly expressed in terms of an inherently multiscale therapeutic intervention, or the 'farming' of pathophysiology within the interpenetrating, shifting, global broadcasts of the human cognome. This will, in fact, be the central thrust of Chapter 10. The next few chapters, however, provide perspectives on, and examples of, the methodology introduced here.

3.6   Refining the Model

Phase transitions

As Feynman (2000) argues, information is simply another form of free energy, and the information in a message can be measured by the free energy needed to erase it. But there are subtleties. To reiterate, information sources are inherently irreversible dynamic systems, even on a microscopic scale, with few and short reversible palindromes: again, in spoken or written English, the short sequence 'the' has much higher probability than its time reversal 'eht'. There is no local reversibility, and adaptation of methods from nonequilibrium statistical mechanics or thermodynamics will not be graced with 'Onsager reciprocal relations'.

Another subtlety is that, in spite of the inherently nonequilibrium dynamic nature of an information source, the asymptotic limit theorems defining information source uncertainty appear to permit 'nonequilibrium equilibria' in a certain sense.

Assume a monotonic increasing measure of available free energy intensity M, $Q(\kappa M), Q(0) = 0$ where κ is again an appropriate inverse energy scaling constant. Further assume that possible generalized cognitive trajectories are constrained by the availability of energy resources, so that the probability of an (inherently irreversible and highly dynamic) information source associated with a groupoid element G_j defined by cognitive process, at a fixed $Q(\kappa M)$, is given, in a first approximation, by the standard expression for the Gibbs distribution

$$P[H_{G_j}] = \frac{\exp[-H_{G_j}/Q]}{\sum_i \exp[-H_{G_i}/Q]}. \tag{3.17}$$

The Gibbs distribution appears to be not really appropriate for systems evolving in an open manner, and it is possible to generalize the treatment somewhat, using an adiabatic approximation in which the dynamics remain 'close enough' to a form in which the mathematical theory can work, adapting standard phase transition formalism for transitions between adiabatic realms. In particular, rather than using exponential terms, one might well use any functional form $f(H_{Gi}, Q)$ such that the sum over i converges.

In essence, however, adopting an information source perspective on cognitive process implicitly incorporates the possibility of 'nonequilibrium equilibria' in the sense of Eldredge and Gould (1972).

The 'E-property' of Khinchin (1957) permits division of paths into high and low probability sets and implies the limiting relation $\lim_{n\to\infty} \log[N(n)]/n = H$ and its variants for all high probability paths generated by an ergodic information source. This allows imposition of a powerful regularity onto inherently nonequilibrium information processes.

The partition function-analog of this system is

$$Z_G(Q) = \sum_i \exp[-H_{G_i}/Q]. \tag{3.18}$$

Now define a 'groupoid free energy', F_G, *constructed over the full set of possible trajectories as constrained by available free energy intensity*, as

$$\exp[-F_G/Q] \equiv \sum_i \exp[-H_{G_i}/Q], \tag{3.19}$$

so that

$$F_G(Q) = -Q\log[Z_G(Q)]. \tag{3.20}$$

This is to be taken as a Morse function, in the sense of the Mathematical Appendix. Other – essentially similar – Morse functions may perhaps be defined on this system, having a more 'natural' interpretation from information theory.

Argument is, again, by abduction from statistical physics (Landau and Lifshitz, 2007; Pettini, 2007). The Morse function F_G is constrained by free energy availability in a manner that allows application of Landau's theory of punctuated phase transition in terms of groupoid, rather than group, symmetries.

Recall, again, Landau's perspective on phase transition (Pettini, 2007): certain physical phase transitions take place in the context of a significant symmetry change, with one phase being more symmetric than the other. A symmetry is lost in the transition, i.e., spontaneous symmetry breaking. The greatest possible set of symmetries being that of the Hamiltonian describing the energy states. Usually, states accessible at lower temperatures lack the symmetries available at higher temperatures, so that the lower temperature state is less symmetric, and transitions can be highly punctuated.

Here, the dependence of cognitive process on the availability of metabolic free energy is characterized in terms of groupoid, rather than group, symmetries, and the argument by abduction is essentially similar: Increasing availability of free energy intensity – rising $Q(\kappa M)$ – will allow richer interactions between the basic information sources, and will do so in a highly punctuated manner, as in Eldredge and Gould (1972).

Kadanoff theory

Given F_G as a free energy analog, what are the transitions between adiabatic realms? Suppose, in classic manner, it is possible to define a characteristic 'length', say r, on the system, as more fully described below. It is then possible to define renormalization symmetries in terms of the 'clumping' transformation, so that, for clumps of size R, in an external 'field' of strength J (that can be set to 0 in the limit), one can write, in the usual manner (e.g., Wilson, 1971)

$$F_G[Q(R), J(R)] = f(R)F_G[Q(1), J(1)]$$
$$\chi(Q(R), J(R)) = \frac{\chi(Q(1), J(1))}{R}, \tag{3.21}$$

where χ is a characteristic correlation length.

As described in the Mathematical Appendix, following Wilson (1971), very many 'biological' renormalizations, $f(R)$, are possible that lead to a number of quite different universality classes for phase transition. Indeed, a 'universality class tuning' can be used as a tool for large-scale regulation of the system (Wallace, 2005).

In order to define the metric r, impose a topology on the system, so that, near a particular 'language' A defining some H_G there is (in an appropriate sense) an open set U of closely similar languages $\hat{A}$, such that $A, \hat{A} \subset U$.

Since the information sources are 'similar', for all pairs of languages $A, \hat{A}$ in U, it is possible to:

1. Create an embedding alphabet which includes all symbols allowed to both of them.

2. Define an information-theoretic distortion measure in that extended, joint alphabet between any high probability (grammatical and syntactical) paths in A and $\hat{A}$, written as $d(Ax, \hat{A}x)$ (Cover and Thomas, 2006). Note that these languages do not interact in this approximation.

3. Define a metric on U, for example,

$$r(A, \hat{A}) = |\lim \frac{\int_{A,\hat{A}} d(Ax, \hat{A}x)}{\int_{A,A} d(Ax, A\hat{x})} - 1|, \tag{3.22}$$

using an appropriate integration limit argument over the high probability paths. Note that the integration in the denominator is over different paths within A itself, while in the numerator it is between different paths in A and $\hat{A}$. Consideration suggests r is indeed a formal metric.

Clearly, other approaches to metric construction on U seem possible, as are other approaches to renormalization.

Nonergodic information sources

The ergodic nature of an information source is a generalization of the law of large numbers and implies that the long-time averages can be closely approximated by averages across the probability spaces of those sources. For non-ergodic information sources, a function, $\mathcal{J}(x_n)$, of each path $x_n \rightarrow x$, may be defined, such that $\lim_{n \rightarrow \infty} \mathcal{J}(x_n) = \mathcal{J}(x)$, but $\mathcal{J}$ will not in general be given by the simple cross-sectional laws-of-large numbers analogs above (Khinchin, 1957).

Let $s \equiv d(x, \hat{x})$ for high probability paths x and $\hat{x}$, where d is a distortion measure, as described in Cover and Thomas (2006). For 'nearly' ergodic systems one might use something of the form

$$\mathcal{J}(\hat{x}) \approx \mathcal{J}(x) + sd\mathcal{J}/ds|_{s=0} \tag{3.23}$$

for s sufficiently small. The idea is to take a distortion measure as a kind of Finsler metric, imposing a resulting 'global' structure over an appropriate class of non-ergodic information sources. One question obviously revolves around what properties are metric-independent, in much the same manner as the rate distortion theorem.

These heuristics can be made more precise: take a set of 'high probability' paths $x_n \rightarrow x$.

Suppose, for all such x, there is an open set, U, containing x, on which the following conditions hold:

1. For all paths $\hat{x}_n \rightarrow \hat{x} \in U$, a distortion measure $s_n \equiv d_U(x_n, \hat{x}_n)$ exists.

2. For each path $x_n \rightarrow x$ in U there exists a pathwise invariant function $\mathcal{J}(x_n) \rightarrow \mathcal{J}(x)$, in the sense of Khinchin (1957, p.72). While such a function will almost always exist, only in the case of an ergodic information source can it be identified as an 'entropy' in the usual sense.

3. A function $F_U(s_n, n) \equiv f_n \rightarrow f$ exists, for example,

$$f_n = s_n, \log[s_n]/n, s_n/n, \tag{3.24}$$

and so on.

4. The limit

$$\lim_{n \rightarrow \infty} \frac{\mathcal{J}(x_n) - \mathcal{J}(\hat{x}_n)}{f_n} \equiv \nabla_F \mathcal{J}|_x \tag{3.25}$$

exists and is finite.

Under such conditions, standard global atlas/manifold constructions are possible. Again, $\mathcal{J}$ is not simply given by the usual expressions for source uncertainty if the source is not ergodic, and the phase transition development may be correspondingly more complicated. Restriction to high probability paths simplifies matters considerably, although precisely characterizing them may be difficult, requiring extension of the Shannon–McMillan theorem and its rate distortion generalization.

An essential question is under what circumstances this differential treatment for 'almost' ergodic information sources permits something very much like Khinchin's (1957, p. 54) 'E property' enabling classification of paths into a small set of high probability and a vastly larger set of vanishingly small probability (Khinchin, 1957, p. 74).

Chapter 4

AN EVOLUTIONARY EXCURSION

4.1 Introduction

The formalism developed in the first three chapters is remarkably powerful, and it is worth examining an extension of it to other biological information sources. In particular, it is possible to reframe some current controversies in evolutionary theory from these perspectives.

Richard Lewontin's (2010) review of the book *What Darwin Got Wrong* by Fodor and Piattelli-Palmarini (2010) neatly summarizes the predominant evolutionary paradigm, the 'Modern Synthesis'. As Lewontin puts it:

> The modern skeletal formulation of evolution by natural selection consists of [several] principles that provide a purely mechanical basis for evolutionary change, stripped of its metaphorical elements:
>
> **1. The principle of variation: among individuals in a population there is variation in form, physiology, and behavior.**
>
> **2. The principle of heredity: offspring resemble their parents more than they resemble unrelated individuals.**
>
> **3. The principle of differential reproduction: in a given environment, some forms are more likely to survive and produce more offspring than other forms...**
>
> **4. The principle of mutation: new heritable variation is constantly occurring.**

Tellingly, Lewontin asserts "The trouble with this outline is that ...[t]here is an immense amount of biology that is missing".

The synthesis itself, minus that immense amount of biology, has been formalized, and hence frozen, into the elaborate apparatus of mathematical population genetics that some find quite elegant (e.g., Ewens, 2004). But mathematical fashion – elegance, after all, is in the eye of the beholder – is not quite the same as science.

The omission of the role of embedding environment in the development of organisms (e.g., epigenetic effects such as heritable stress-induced gene methylation) and the omission of other interactions between organism and embedding environment (e.g., niche construction *sensu* Odling-Smee *et al.*, 2003) – severely limits the biological relevance of that synthesis. Here, following Wallace and Wallace (2008, 2009) and Wallace *et al.* (2009), we will describe genes, environment, and gene expression, in terms of information sources that interact and affect each other through a broadly coevolutionary crosstalk having quasi-stable 'resilience' modes in the sense of Holling (1973, 1992).

This implies, among other things, that internal dynamics, for example the 'large deviations' described in Wallace and Wallace (2008), can trigger ecosystem shifts that, in turn, create selection pressure on organisms. The aerobic transition seems a most telling example. External factors may also trigger punctuated ecosystem shifts that can entrain organisms: volcanism, meteor strikes, ice ages, and the like.

But the story doesn't end with niche construction, epigenetics, or catastrophe.

Sun and Caetano-Anolles (2008) claim evidence for deep evolutionary patterns is embedded in tRNA phylogenies, calculated from trees reconstructed from analyses of data from several hundred tRNA molecules. They argue that an observed lack of correlation between ancestries of amino acid charging and encoding indicates the separate discoveries of these functions and reflects independent histories of recruitment. These histories were, in their view, probably curbed by co-options and important take-overs during early diversification of the living world. That is, disjoint evolutionary patterns were associated with evolution of amino acid specificity and codon identity, indicating that co-options and take-overs embedded perhaps in horizontal gene transfer affected differently the amino acid charging and codon identity functions. These results, they claim, support a strand symmetric ancient world in which tRNA had both a genetic and a functional role (Rodin and Rodin, 2008).

Clearly, 'co-options' and 'take-overs' are, perhaps, most easily explained as products of a prebiotic serial endosymbiosis, instantiated by a Red Queen between significantly, perhaps radically, different precursor chemical systems.

Witzany (2009) also takes a broadly similar 'language' approach to the transfer of heritage information between different kinds of proto-organisms. In that paper he reviews a massive literature, arguing that not only rRNA, but also tRNA and the processing of the primary transcript into the pre-mRNA and the mature mRNA seem to be remnants of viral infection events that did not kill their host, but transferred phenotypic competences to their host and changed both the genetic identity of the host organism and the identity of the former infectious viral swarms. His 'biocommunication' viewpoint investigates both communication within and among cells, tissues, organs and organisms as sign-mediated interactions, and nucleotide sequences as code, that is, language-like text.

Thus, editing genetic text sequences requires, similar to the signaling codes between cells, tissues, and organs, biotic agents that are competent in correct sign use. Otherwise, neither communication processes nor nucleotide sequence generation or recombination can function. From his perspective, DNA is not only an information storing archive, but a life habitat for nucleic acid language-using RNA agents of viral or subviral descent able to carry out almost error-free editing of nucleotide sequences according to systematic rules of grammar and syntax.

Koonin et al. (2006) and Vetsigian et al. (2006) take a roughly similar tack, without, however, invoking biocommunication: Koonin et al. postulate a Virus World that has coexisted with cellular organisms from deep evolutionary time, and Vetsigian et al. suggest a long period of vesicle crosstalk symbiosis driving standardization of genetic codes across competing populations, leading to a 'Darwinian transition' representing path-dependent lock-in of genetic codes.

In particular, before the lock-in of the precursor of the current genetic code (e.g., Tlusty, 2007, 2008; Wallace, 2010), vesicle structure may have been rather more plastic than today, permitting analogs to gene transfer between quite different prebiotic organisms.

Synthesizing these considerations generates a fifth principle:

5. The principle of environmental interaction: individuals and groups engage in powerful, often punctuated, dynamic mutual relations with their embedding environments that may include the exchange of heritage material between markedly different organisms.

The central step is reexpression of some familiar biological phenomena as information sources, leading to a formal mathematical structure that expresses these extensions.

4.2   Ecosystems as Information Sources

Consider a simplistic picture of an elementary predator/prey ecosystem. Let X represent the appropriately scaled number of 'predators', Y the scaled number of 'prey', t the time, and ω a parameter defining their interaction. The model assumes that the ecologically dominant relation is an interaction between predator and prey, so that $dX/dt = \omega Y$ and $dY/dt = -\omega X$.

Thus, the predator population grows proportionately to the prey population, and the prey declines proportionately to the predator population.

Differentiating the first and using the second equation gives the simple relation $d^2X/dt^2 + \omega^2 X = 0$, having the solution $X(t) = \sin(\omega t); Y(t) = \cos(\omega t)$. Thus, $X(t)^2 + Y(t)^2 = \sin^2(\omega t) + \cos^2(\omega t) \equiv 1$.

In the two-dimensional phase space defined by $X(t)$ and $Y(t)$, the system traces out an endless, circular trajectory in time, representing the out-of-phase sinusoidal oscillations of the predator and prey populations.

Divide the $X - Y$ phase space into two components, the simplest coarse-graining, calling the halfplane to the left of the vertical Y-axis A and that to the right B. This system, over units of the period $1/(2\pi\omega)$, traces out a stream of As and Bs having a single very precise grammar and syntax: $ABABABAB...$

Many other such statements might be conceivable, e.g.,

$$AAAAA..., BBBBB..., AAABAAAB..., ABAABAAAB...,$$

and so on, but, of the obviously infinite number of possibilities, only one is actually observed, is 'grammatical': $ABABABAB....$

More complex dynamical system models, incorporating diffusional drift around deterministic solutions, or even very elaborate systems of complicated stochastic differential equations, having various domains of attraction, that is, different sets of grammars, can be described by analogous symbolic dynamics (Beck and Schlogl, 1993, Ch. 3).

Rather than taking symbolic dynamics as a simplification of more exact analytic or stochastic approaches, it is possible to generalize symbolic dynamics to a more comprehensive information dynamics. Ecosystems may not have identifiable sets of stochastic dynamic equations like noisy, nonlinear mechanical clocks, but, under appropriate coarse-graining, they may still have recognizable sets of grammar and syntax over the long term. For example, the turn of the seasons in a temperate climate, for many natural communities, looks remarkably the same year after year: the ice melts, the migrating birds return, the trees bud, the grass grows, plants and animals reproduce, high summer arrives, the foliage turns, the birds leave, frost, snow, the rivers freeze, and so on.

Suppose it possible to empirically characterize an ecosystem at a given time t by observations of both habitat parameters such as temperature and rainfall, and numbers of various plant and animal species.

Traditionally, one can then calculate a cross-sectional species diversity index at time t using an information or entropy metric of the form

$$H = -\sum_{j=1}^{M} (n_j/N) \log[(n_j/N)],$$

$$N \equiv \sum_{j=1}^{M} n_j,$$

where n_j is the number of observed individuals of species j and N is the total number of individuals of all species observed (e.g., Pielou, 1977).

This is not the approach to be taken here. Quite the contrary, in fact. Suppose it possible to coarse-grain the ecosystem at time t according to some appropriate partition of the phase space in which each division A_j represents a particular range of numbers of each possible species in the ecosystem, along with associated parameters such as temperature, rainfall, and the like. What is of particular interest here is not cross-sectional structure, but rather longitudinal paths, that is, ecosystem statements of the form $x_n = \{A_0, A_1, ..., A_n\}$ defined in terms of some natural time unit of the system. Thus, n corresponds to an appropriate characteristic time unit T, so that $t = T, 2T, ..., nT$.

To reiterate, unlike the traditional use of information theory in ecology, the central interest is in the *serial correlations along paths*, and not at all in the cross-sectional entropy calculated for of a single element of a path.

Let $N(n)$ be the number of possible paths of length n that are consistent with the underlying grammar and syntax of the appropriately coarse-grained ecosystem: spring leads to summer, autumn, winter, back to spring, etc., but never something of the form spring to autumn to summer to winter in a temperate ecosystem.

The fundamental assumptions are that – for this chosen coarse-graining – $N(n)$, the number of possible grammatical paths, is much smaller than the total number of paths possible, and that, in the limit of (relatively) large n, $H = \lim_{n\to\infty} \log[N(n)]/n$ both exists and is independent of path, as in the argument leading to Eq. (1.1).

To reiterate, this is a critical foundation to, and limitation on, the modeling strategy and its range of strict applicability, but is, in a sense, fairly general since it is independent of the details of the serial correlations along a path.

Again, these conditions are the essence of the parallel with parametric statistics. Systems for which the assumptions are not true will require special nonparametric approaches. It can be argued, however, that, as for parametric statistical inference, the methodology will prove robust in that many systems will sufficiently fulfill the essential criteria.

This being said, not all possible ecosystem coarse-grainings are likely to work, and different such divisions, even when appropriate, might well lead to different descriptive quasi-languages for the ecosystem of interest. The example of Markov models is relevant. The essential Markov assumption is that the probability of a transition from one state at time T to another at time $T + \Delta T$ depends only on the state at T, and not at all on the history by which that state was reached. If changes within the interval of length ΔT are plastic, or path dependent, then attempts to model the system as a Markov process *within* the natural interval ΔT will fail, even though the model works quite well for phenomena separated by natural intervals.

Thus, empirical identification of relevant coarse-grainings for which this body of theory will work is clearly not trivial, and may, in fact, constitute the hard scientific core of the matter.

This is not, however, a new difficulty in ecosystem theory. Holling (1992), for example, explores the linkage of ecosystems across scales, finding that mesoscale structures – what might correspond to the neighborhood in a human community – are ecological keystones in space, time, and population, which drive process and pattern at both smaller and larger scales and levels of organization.

Levin (1989) argues that there is no single correct scale of observation: the insights from any investigation are contingent on the choice of scales. Pattern is neither a property of the system alone nor of the observer, but of an interaction between them. Pattern exists at all levels and at all scales, and recognition of this multiplicity of scales is fundamental to describing and understanding ecosystems. In his view there can be no 'correct' level of aggregation: one must recognize explicitly the multiplicity of scales within ecosystems, and develop a perspective that looks across scales and that builds on a multiplicity of models rather than seeking the single 'correct' one.

Given an appropriately chosen coarse-graining, whose selection in many cases will be the difficult and central trick of scientific art, suppose it possible to define joint and conditional probabilities for different ecosystem paths, having the form $P(A_0, A_1, ..., A_n), P(A_n|A_0, ..., A_{n-1})$, such that appropriate joint and conditional Shannon uncertainties can be defined on them. For paths of length two these would be of the form

$$H(X_1, X_2) \equiv -\sum_j \sum_k P(A_j, A_k) \log[P(A_j, A_k)]$$

and

$$H(X_1|X_2) \equiv -\sum_j \sum_k P(A_j, A_k) \log[P(A_j|A_k)],$$

where the X_j represent the stochastic processes generating the respective paths of interest.

The essential content of the Shannon–McMillan theorem is that, for a large class of systems characterized as information sources, a kind of law-of-large numbers exists in the limit of very long paths, so that, again, the results of Eq. (1.2) hold:

$$H[X] = \lim_{n\to\infty} \frac{\log[N(n)]}{n} =$$

$$\lim_{n\to\infty} H(X_n|X_0, ..., X_{n-1}) =$$

$$\lim_{n\to\infty} \frac{H(X_0, X_1, ..., X_n)}{n+1}.$$

Taking the definitions of Shannon uncertainties as above, and arguing backwards from the latter two equations, it is indeed possible to recover the first, and divide the set of all possible temporal paths of our ecosystem into two subsets, one very small, containing the grammatically correct, and hence highly probable paths, that can be called 'meaningful', and a much larger set of vanishingly low probability (Khinchin, 1957).

4.3 Genetic Heritage

Adami *et al.* (2000) make a case for reinterpreting the Darwinian transmission of genetic heritage in terms of a formal information process. They assert that genomic complexity can be identified with the amount of information a sequence stores about its environment: genetic complexity can be defined in a consistent information-theoretic manner. In their view, information cannot exist in a vacuum and must be instantiated. For biological systems, information is instantiated, in part, by DNA. To some extent it is the blueprint of an organism and thus information about its own structure. More specifically, it is a blueprint of how to build an organism that can best survive in its native environment, and pass on that information to its progeny. Adami *et al.* assert that an organism's DNA thus is not only a 'book' about the organism, but also a book about the environment it lives in, including the species with which it coevolves. They identify the complexity of genomes by the amount of information they encode about the world in which they have evolved.

Ofria *et al.* (2003) continue in the same direction and argue that genomic complexity can be defined rigorously within standard information theory as the information the genome of an organism contains about its environment. From the point of view of information theory, it is convenient to view Darwinian evolution on the molecular level as a collection of information transmission channels, subject to a number of constraints. In these channels, they state, the organism's genome codes for the information (a message) to be transmitted from progenitor to offspring, subject to noise from an imperfect replication process and multiple sources of contingency. Information theory is concerned with analyzing the properties of such channels, how much information can be transmitted and how the rate of perfect information transmission of such a channel can be maximized.

Adami and Cerf (2000) argue, using simple models of genetic structure, that the information content, or complexity, of a genomic string by itself (without referring to an environment) is a meaningless concept and a change in environment (catastrophic or otherwise) generally leads to a pathological reduction in complexity.

The transmission of genetic information is thus a contextual matter involving operation of an information source that, according to this perspective, must interact with embedding (ecosystem) structures. Such interaction is, as shown below, often highly punctuated, modulated by mesoscale ecosystem transitions via a generalization of the Baldwin effect akin to stochastic resonance i.e., a 'mesoscale resonance' (Wallace and Wallace, 2008, 2009).

4.4   Gene Expression

Wallace and Wallace (2008, 2009), following the footsteps of Cohen and Harel (2007) and O'Nuallain (2008), argue at some formal length that a 'cognitive paradigm' is needed to understand gene expression, much as Atlan and Cohen (1998) invoke a cognitive paradigm for the immune system.

Cohen and Harel (2007) assert that gene expression is a reactive system that calls our attention to its emergent properties, i.e., behaviors that, taken as a whole, are not expressed by any one of the lower scale components that comprise it: cellular processes react to both internal and external signals to produce diverse tissues internally, and diverse general phenotypes across various scales of space, time, and population, all from a single set or relatively narrow distribution of genes.

The essential point, from the perspective of this chapter, is that a broad class of cognitive phenomena can be characterized in terms of a dual information source that can interact with other such sources. As discussed above, Atlan and Cohen (1998) argue that the essence of cognition is comparison of a perceived external signal with an internal, learned picture of the world, and then, upon that comparison, the choice of one response from a much larger repertoire of possible responses. Such reduction in uncertainty inherently carries information, and it is possible to make a very general model of this process as an information source.

Cognitive pattern recognition-and-selected response, as conceived here, proceeds by convoluting an incoming external 'sensory' signal with an internal 'ongoing activity' – including, but not limited to, the learned picture of the world – and, at some point, triggering an appropriate action based on a decision that the pattern of sensory activity requires a response. It is not necessary to specify how the pattern recognition system is trained, and hence possible to adopt a weak model, regardless of learning paradigm, that can itself be more formally described by the rate distortion theorem. Fulfilling Atlan and Cohen's criterion of meaning-from-response, a language's contextual meaning can be defined entirely in terms of system output.

The model follows the arguments of Section 1.3.

It is thus possible to define an ergodic information source $\mathbf{X}$ associated with stochastic variates X_j having joint and conditional probabilities such that appropriate joint and conditional Shannon uncertainties satisfy the relations above. This information source is, again, taken as dual to the ergodic cognitive process.

Different quasi-languages will be defined by different divisions of the total universe of possible responses into various pairs of sets B_0 and B_1 as in Section 1.3. Like the use of different distortion measures in the rate distortion theorem, however, it seems obvious that the underlying dynamics will all be qualitatively similar.

It is worth noting that dividing the full set of possible responses into the sets B_0 and B_1 may itself require higher order cognitive decisions by another module or modules, suggesting the necessity of choice within a more or less broad set of possible quasi-languages. This would directly reflect the need to shift gears according to the different challenges faced by the organism or organic subsystem. A critical problem then becomes the choice of a normal zero-mode language among a very large set of possible languages representing accessible excited states. This is a fundamental matter mirroring, for isolated cognitive systems, the resilience arguments applicable to more conventional ecosystems, that is, the possibility of more than one zero state to a cognitive system. Identification of an excited state as the zero mode becomes, then, a kind of generalized autoimmune disorder that can be triggered by linkage with external ecological information sources representing various kinds of structured stress. This will be a frequently recurring theme in these chapters.

In sum, meaningful paths – creating an inherent grammar and syntax – have been defined entirely in terms of system response, as Atlan and Cohen propose.

4.5   Interacting Information Sources

It is possible to model the interaction of these information sources: embedding environment, genetic heritage (possibly across different organisms), and cognitive gene expression, using a straightforward formalism similar to that invoked both for nonequilibrium thermodynamics and traditional studies of coevolution (e.g., Deikmann and Law, 1996).

The argument recapitulates much of Chapter 3, but in evolutionary language:

Consider a set of crosstalk measures, I_j, between a set of information sources. Use the measures $I_j, j \neq m$ *as parameters for each of the others,* writing $I_m = I_m(K_1...K_s, ...I_j...), j \neq m$, where the K_s represent other relevant parameters.

Now segregate the I_j according to their relative rates of change. Cognitive gene expression would be among the most rapid, followed by ecosystem dynamics and evolutionary selection.

The dynamics of such a system becomes a recursive network of stochastic differential equations similar to those used to study many other highly parallel dynamic structures (Wymer, 1997).

Letting the K_j and I_m all be represented as parameters Q^j, (with the caveat that I_m not depend on itself), one can define a 'disorder' measure analogous to entropy in nonequilibrium thermodynamics, following the arguments of Chapter 3, $S_I^m \equiv I_m - \sum_i Q^i \partial I_m / \partial Q^i$ to obtain a complicated recursive system of phenomenological 'Onsager' stochastic differential equations,

$$dQ_t^j = \sum_i [L_{j,i}(t, ...\partial S_I^m / \partial Q^i ...) dt + \sigma_{j,i}(t, ...\partial S_I^m / \partial Q^i ...) dB_t^i]$$

$$= L_j(t, Q^1, ..., Q^n) dt + \sum_i \sigma(t, Q^1, .., Q^n) dB_t^i, \quad (4.1)$$

where terms have been collected and expressed as both the Is and the external Ks using the same Q^j, and the gradient of the S^m with respect to the Q^i represents the analog to 'thermodynamic force' in a physical system.

The index m ranges over the crosstalk and we could allow different kinds of 'noise' dB_t^i, having particular forms of quadratic variation which may, in fact, represent a projection of environmental factors under something like a rate distortion manifold (Glazebrook and Wallace, 2009a, b).

The origin of this approach lies in the formal similarity between the expression for free energy density and information source uncertainty, explored earlier.

The argument of Section 3.1 carries through:

1. Setting the system of Eqs. (4.1) equal to zero and solving for stationary points gives attractor states since the noise terms preclude unstable equilibria.

2. This system may converge to limit cycle or pseudorandom 'strange attractor' behaviors in which the system seems to chase its tail endlessly within a limited venue – the traditional Red Queen.

3. What is converged to in both cases is not a simple state or limit cycle of states. Rather it is an equivalence class, or set of them, of highly dynamic information sources coupled by mutual interaction through crosstalk. Thus 'stability' in this structure represents particular patterns of ongoing dynamics rather than some identifiable static configuration.

It is of some interest to compare these results to the work of Diekmann and Law (1996), who invoke evolutionary game dynamics to obtain a first order canonical equation for coevolutionary systems having the form

$$ds_i/dt = K_i(s) \partial W_i(s_i', s)|_{s_i' = s_i}. \quad (4.2)$$

The s_i, with $i = 1, ..., N$, denote adaptive trait values in a community comprising N species. The $W_i(s_i', s)$ are measures of fitness of individuals with trait values s_i' in the environment determined by the resident trait values s, and the $K_i(s)$ are non-negative coefficients, possibly distinct for each species, that scale the rate of evolutionary change. Adaptive dynamics of this kind have frequently been postulated, based either on the notion of a hill-climbing process on an adaptive landscape or some other sort of plausibility argument.

When this equation is set equal to zero, so there is no time dependence, one obtains what are characterized as 'evolutionary singularities' or stationary points.

Diekmann and Law contend that their formal derivation of this equation satisfies four critical requirements:

1. The evolutionary process needs to be considered in a coevolutionary context.

2. A proper mathematical theory of evolution should be dynamical.

3. The coevolutionary dynamics ought to be underpinned by a microscopic theory.

4. The evolutionary process has important stochastic elements.

Equation (4.1) above, in its evolutionary incarnation adopted here, is similar, although reached through a very different route, allowing elaborate patterns of phase transition punctuation in a highly natural manner (Wallace and Wallace, 2008). Again, it is possible to invoke the large deviation arguments of Champagnat *et al.* (2006), leading to Eq. (3.5).

These considerations lead very much in the direction of an evolutionary version of Eq. (3.3), invoked above in Eq. (4.1), but again seen as subject to internally driven large deviations that are themselves described as information sources, providing $\mathcal{I}$ crosstalk parameters that can trigger punctuated shifts between quasi-stable modes, in addition to resilience transitions driven by 'catastrophic' external events or the exchange of heritage information between different classes of organisms.

Equation (4.1) provides a very general statistical model that combines principle (5) – in concert with the possibility of large deviations – with earlier theory.

Indeed, the direct inclusion of large deviation regularities within the context of the statistical model of Eq. (4.1) suggests that other factors that can be characterized in terms of information sources may be directly included within the formalism. Section 6.1 of Wallace *et al.*, (2009), for example, explores the impact of culture, taken as a generalized language, on the evolution of human pathogens. The methodology thus provides a straightforward means of incorporating the evolutionary effects of animal traditions, as described by Avital and Jablonka (2000).

The basic statistical model is illustrated by Fig. 4.1, an evolutionary version of Fig. 3.1, for a 'fast' time, 'small' scale process. Here, two quasi-equilibria are characterized by diffusive drift about their singularities in a two-dimensional system, but are coupled by a highly structured large deviation connecting them. The pattern most obviously encompasses the punctuated equilibrium of Eldredge and Gould (1972).

Figure 4.2 expands the system of Fig. 4.1 to 'slow' time, 'large' scale, so that the large deviations of Fig. 4.1 are seen as, in essence, variation about a single 'larger' singularity. This latter structure could account for the observations of Gomez et al. (2010) who show that, as with other niche components, ecological interactions are evolutionarily conserved, suggesting a shared pattern in the organization of biological systems through evolutionary time that is particularly mediated by marked conservation of ecological interactions among taxa.

4.6 Conclusions

It is possible to reexpress ecosystem dynamics, genetic heritage, and (cognitive) gene expression producing phenotypes that interact with the embedding ecosystem, all in terms of interacting information sources. This instantiates principle (5) in Section 4.1, producing a system of stochastic differential equations closely analogous to those used to describe more traditional coevolutionary phenomena, subject to punctuated resilience shifts driven both by internal large deviations and large-scale external perturbations.

That is, environments affect living things, and living things affect their environments. Cyanobacteria, for example, created the aerobic transition, greatly changing the very atmosphere of the planet. Organisms can, more locally, engage in niche construction that changes the local environment as profoundly. Environments select phenotypes that, in a sense, select environments. Genes record the result, as does the embedding landscape. The system coevolves as a unit, with sudden, complicated transitions between the quasiequilibria defined by setting the Eq. (4.1) to zero, the evolutionary version of Eq. (3.3).

To reiterate, these transitions can be driven by internal 'large deviation' dynamics, as the aerobic transition, or by external events, volcanic erup-

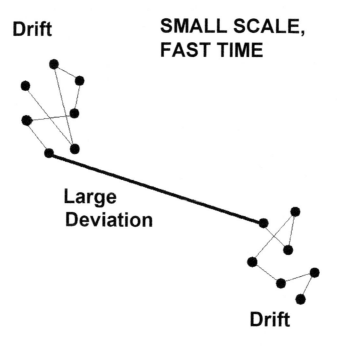

Fig. 4.1 'Small' scale, 'fast' time behavior of the system obtained by setting Eq. (4.1) to zero. Diffusive drift about a quasi-equilibrium is interrupted by a highly structured large deviation leading to another quasi-equilibrium, in the pattern of punctuated equilibrium of Eldredge and Gould. Compare with Fig. 3.1.

tions or meteor strikes, and so on. Ecosystem resilience shifts entrain the evolution of individual organisms that, in turn, drive ecosystem resilience transitions.

Enlargement of scale, however, can produce a model of the conservation of ecological interactions across the tree of life.

Thus the introduction of principle (5) to the Modern Synthesis generates a complex model, perhaps best characterized by the term 'evolution of ecosystems'. The essential point is that the Modern Synthesis now requires modernizing, recognizing the importance and ubiquity of a mutual interaction with the embedding ecosystem that includes the possibility of the exchange of heritage information between different classes of organisms.

This work outlines a 'natural' means for implementing such a program, based on the asymptotic limit theorems of communication theory that pro-

LARGE SCALE, SLOW TIME

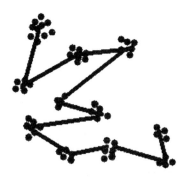

Fig. 4.2 'Large' scale, 'slow' time enlargement of Fig. 4.1, showing the conservation of ecological interactions across deep evolutionary time as variation about a single, larger, singularity.

vide necessary conditions constraining the dynamics of all systems producing or exchanging information, in the same sense that the central limit theorem provides constraints on systems that involve sums of stochastic variates. That is, it provides the basis for a new set of statistical tools useful in the study of ecological and evolutionary phenomena. Statistics, however, is not science, and the fundamental problems of data acquisition, ordination, and interpretation remain.

Chapter 5

EXAMPLE: MENTAL DISORDERS

5.1 Introduction

The multilevel nested cognition model constructed in the earlier chapters may provide some insight into current controversies regarding mental disorders. Indeed, human mental disorders are not well understood, and their study provides a difficult example for theories of disease heritability. Official classifications as the *Diagnostic and Statistical Manual of Mental Disorders - fourth edition*, (DSM-IV, 1994), the standard descriptive nosology in the US, have even been characterized as 'prescientific' by P. Gilbert (2001) and others. Johnson-Laird *et al.* (2006) claim that current knowledge about psychological illnesses is comparable to the medical understanding of epidemics in the early 19th century. Physicians realized then that cholera, for example, was a specific disease, killing about a third of the people whom it infected. What they disagreed about was the cause, the pathology, and the communication of the disease. Similarly, according to Johnson-Laird *et al.*, most medical professionals these days realize that psychological illnesses occur (cf. DSM-IV), but they disagree about their cause and pathology. Notwithstanding DSM-IV, Johnson-Laird *et al.* doubt whether any satisfactory *a priori* definition of psychological illness can exist because it is a matter for theory to elucidate.

Atmanspacher (2006) argues that formal theory of high-level cognitive process is itself at a point similar to that of physics 400 years ago, in that the basic entities, and the relations between them, have yet to be delineated.

More generally, simple arguments from genetic determinism regarding mental disorders fail, in part because of a draconian population bottleneck that, early in our species' history, resulted in an overall genetic diversity less than that observed within and between contemporary chimpanzee subgroups. Manolio *et al.* (2009) describe this conundrum more generally in terms of 'finding the missing heritability of complex diseases'. They observe, for example, that at least 40 loci have been associated with human height, a classic complex trait with an estimated heritability of about 80%, yet they explain only about 5% of phenotype variance despite studies of tens of thousands of people. This result, they find, is typical across a broad range of supposedly heritable diseases, and call for extending beyond current genome-wide assoication approaches to illuminate the genetics of complex diseases and enhance its potential to enable effective disease prevention or treatment.

Arguments from psychosocial stress fare better (e.g., Brown *et al.*, 1973; Dohrenwend and Dohrenwend, 1974; Eaton, 1978), particularly for depression (e.g., Risch *et al.*, 2009), but are affected by the apparently complex and contingent developmental paths determining the onset of schizophrenia, dementias, psychoses, and so forth, some of which may be triggered *in utero* by exposure to infection, low birthweight, or other functional teratogens.

P. Gilbert (2001) suggests an extended evolutionary perspective, in which evolved mechanisms like the 'flight-or-fight' response are inappropriately excited or suppressed, resulting in such conditions as anxiety or posttraumatic stress disorders. Nesse (2000) suggests that depression may represent the dysfunction of an evolutionary adaptation which down-regulates foraging activity in the face of unattainable goals.

Kleinman and Good (1985, p. 492), however, outline something of the cross cultural subtleties affecting the study of depression that seem to argue against any simple evolutionary or genetic interpretation. They state that, when culture is treated as a constant, as is common when studies are conducted in our own society, it is relatively easy to view depression as a biological disorder, triggered by social stressors in the presence of ineffective support, and reflected in a set of symptoms or complaints that map back onto the biological substrate of the disorder. However, they continue, when culture is treated as a significant variable, for example, when the researcher seriously confronts the world of meaning and experience of members of non-Western societies, many of our assumptions about the nature of emotions and illness are cast in sharp relief. Dramatic differences are found across cultures in the social organization, personal experience, and consequences of such emotions as sadness, grief, and anger, of behaviors such as withdrawal or aggression, and of psychological characteristics such as passivity and helplessness or the resort to altered states of consciousness. They are organized differently as psychological realities, communicated in a wide range of idioms, related to quite varied local contexts of power relations, and are interpreted, evaluated, and responded to as fundamentally different meaningful realities. Depressive illness and dysphoria are thus not only interpreted differently in non-Western societies and across cultures; they are *constituted* as fundamentally different forms of social reality.

Since publication of that landmark study, a number of comprehensive overviews support its conclusions, for example, Bebbington (1993), Jenkins, Kleniman and Good (1990), Journal of Clinical Psychiatry (Supplement 13), and Manson (1995). As Marsella (2003) writes, it is now clear that cultural variations exist in the areas of meaning, perceived causes, onset patterns, epidemiology, symptom expression, course, and outcome, variations having important implications for understanding clinical activities including conceptualization, assessment, and therapy.

Kleinman and Cohen (1997) argue forcefully that several myths have become central to psychiatry. The first is that the forms of mental illness everywhere display similar degrees of prevalence. The second is an excessive adherence to a principle known as the pathogenic–pathoplastic dichotomy, which holds that biology is responsible for the underlying structure of a malaise, whereas cultural beliefs shape the specific ways in which a person experiences it. The third myth maintains that various unusual culture-specific disorders whose biological bases are uncertain occur only in exotic places outside the West. In an effort to base psychiatry in 'hard' science and thus raise its status to that of other medical disciplines, psychiatrists have narrowly focused on the biological underpinnings of mental disorders while discounting the importance of such 'soft' variables as culture and socioeconomic status.

Heine (2001) describes an explicit cultural psychology that views the person as containing a set of biological potentials interacting with particular situational contexts that constrain and afford the expression of various constellations of traits and patterns of behavior. He says that, unlike much of personality psychology, cultural psychology focuses on the constraints and affordances inherent to the cultural environment that give shape to those biological potentials. Human nature, from this perspective, is seen as emerging from participation in cultural worlds, and of adapting oneself to the imperatives of cultural directives, meaning that our nature is ultimately that of a cultural being.

Heine describes how cultural psychology does not view culture as a superficial wrapping of the self, or as a framework within which selves interact, but as something that is intrinsic to the self, so that without culture there is no self, only a biological entity deprived of its potential. Individual selves, from Heine's perspective, are inextricably grounded in a configuration of consensual understandings and behavioral customs particular to a given cultural and historical context, so that understanding the self requires an understanding of the culture that sustains it. Heine argues, then, that the process of becoming a self is contingent on individuals interacting with, and seizing meanings from, the cultural environment.

Heine warns that the extreme nature of American individualism means that a psychology based on late 20th century American research not only stands the risk of developing models that are particular to that culture, but of developing an understanding of the self that is peculiar in the context of the world's cultures.

Indeed, as Norenzayan and Heine (2005) point out, for the better part of a hundred years, a considerable controversy has raged within anthropology regarding the degree to which psychological and other human universals do, in fact, actually exist independent of the particularities of culture.

Arnett (2008), in a paper provocatively titled 'The Neglected 95%', similarly argues that US psychological research focuses too narrowly on Americans, who comprise less than 5% of the world's population, and on perhaps another 7% in Western countries. He asserts that the majority of the world's population lives under vastly different conditions, underlying doubts of how representative American psychological research can be, and finds the narrowness of American research to be a consequence of a focus on a philosophy of science that emphasizes fundamental processes and ignores or strips away cultural context.

Henrich *et al.* (2010), in a wide-ranging review, extend the considerations of Norenzayan and Heine, finding that Western, educated, industrialized and democratic (WEIRD) subjects, across domains of visual perception, fairness, categorization, spatial cognition, memory, moral reasoning, and self-concepts, constitute frequent outliers compared with the rest of the species. They conclude that addressing questions of *human* psychology will require tapping broader subject pools.

As Durham (1991) and Richerson and Boyd (2006) explore at some length, humans are endowed with two distinct but interacting heritage systems: genes and culture. Durham (1991), for example, writes that genes and culture constitute two distinct but interacting systems of information inheritance within human populations and information of both kinds has influence, actual or potential, over behaviors, which creates a real and unambiguous symmetry between genes and phenotypes on the one hand, and culture and phenotypes on the other. Genes and culture, in his view, are best represented as two parallel lines or tracks of hereditary influence on phenotypes.

Both genes and culture can be envisioned as generalized languages in that they have recognizable 'grammar' and 'syntax', in the sense of the previous chapters (Wallace, 2005; Wallace and Wallace, 2008, 2009).

More recent work has identified epigenetic heritage mechanisms involving such processes as environmentally induced gene methylation, that can have strong influence across several generations (e.g., Jablonka and Lamb, 1995, 1998; Jabolonka, 2004), and are the subject of intense current research.

There are, it seems, two powerful heritage mechanisms in addition to the genetic where one may perhaps find the 'missing heritability of complex diseases' that Manolio *et al.* seek.

Here, however, the particular interest lies in the phenotypes of madness, and in their relations to genes, culture, and environment.

5.2 Two Classes

Gene–environment interaction

Much recent work in American biological psychiatry has emphasized the search for gene–environment interactions. Caspi and Moffitt (2006), for example, claim that such interactions occur when the effect of exposure to an environmental pathogen on a person's health is conditional on his or her genotype. The first evidence that genotype moderates the capacity of an environmental risk to bring about mental disorders was, according to them, reported in 2002 (Caspi *et al.*, 2002), in a study of the role of genotype in the cycle of violence in maltreated children. Caspi and Moffitt (2006) claim that the gene–environment interaction approach brings opportunities for extending the range and power of neuroscience by introducing opportunities for collaboration between experimental neuroscience and research on gene–environment interactions. Successful collaboration can, in their view, solve the biggest mystery of human psychopathology: how does an environmental factor, external to the person, get inside the nervous system and alter its elements to generate the symptoms of a disordered mind? Concentrating the considerable resources of neuroscience and gene–environment interaction on this question will, they claim, bring discoveries that advance the understanding of mental disorders, and increase the potential to control and prevent them.

One of the most cited of recent studies of gene–environment interactions is, indeed, the work of Caspi *et al.* (2003), who found that genetic variation in the promoter region of the serotonin transporter gene (5-HTTLPR;[OMIM182138]), in interaction with stressful life events, contributes to a predisposition to major depression. As Risch *et al.* (2009) put it, this result was striking and potentially paradigm shifting because numerous previous studies of this same polymorphism, without examining environmental risk factors or life events, had not consistently shown either a strong or replicated association with depression. A subsequent meta-analysis was conducted by Risch *et al.* (2009) that combined data from some 14 studies having a total of 14,250 participants, some 1,769 of whom met criteria for depression.

Risch *et al.* state that most of the participants were white, except for a multiethnic sample in one study, and an Asian sample in another. Contrary to the results of Caspi *et al.* (2003), they found no evidence that the serotonin transporter genotype alone, or in interaction with stressful life events, is associated with an elevated risk of depression.

The Asian study, by J. Kim *et al.* (2007), involved 732 Korean community residents ages 65+, a fair number indeed. Some 88% at baseline did not meet criteria for depression. Kim *et al.*, in contrast with Risch *et al.*, in spite of using 'standard' instruments for both measures of depression and life events (translated into Korean), found a strong statistical trend suggesting that environmental risk of depression is indeed modified by at least two genes, and that gene–environment interactions are found even into old age.

Given the scathing analyses by Arnett, Heine, and Henrich *et al.*, the bitter conflict between the results of Caspi *et al.* (2003) and Risch *et al.* (2009) is in serious danger of becoming simply a culture-bound tempest in a distinctly American teapot.

Gene–culture interaction

The necessity for the inclusion of culture in the operation of fundamental psychological phenomena is emphasized by the observations of Nisbett *et al.* (2001), and others, following the tradition of Markus and Kitayama (1991), regarding profound differences in basic perception between test subjects of Southeast Asian and Western cultural heritage across an broad realm of experiments. East Asian perspectives are characterized as *holistic* and Western as *analytic*. Nisbett *et al.* (2001) find:

1. Social organization directs attention to some aspects of the perceptual field at the expense of others.

2. What is attended to influences metaphysics.

3. Metaphysics guides tacit epistemology, that is, beliefs about the nature of the world and causality.

4. Epistemology dictates the development and application of some cognitive processes at the expense of others.

5. Social organization can directly affect the plausibility of metaphysical assumptions, such as whether causality should be regarded as residing in the field vs. in the object.

6. Social organization and social practice can directly influence the development and use of cognitive processes such as dialectical vs. logical ones.

Nisbett *et al.* (2001) conclude that tools of thought embody a culture's intellectual history, that tools have theories built into them, and that users accept these theories, albeit unknowingly, when they use these tools.

More recently, Masuda and Nisbett (2006) examined cultural variations in change blindness, a phenomenon related to inattentional blindness, and found striking differences between Western and East Asian subjects. They presented participants with still photos and with animated vignettes having changes in focal object information and contextual information. Compared to Americans, East Asians were more sensitive to contextual changes than to focal object changes. These results, they conclude, suggest that there can be cultural variation in what may seem to be basic perceptual processes.

H. Kim *et al.* (2010) have extended this line of work to examine the interaction between genes and culture as determinants of individuals' locus of attention. As the serotonin (5-HT) system has been associated with attentional focus and the ability to adapt to changes in reinforcement, they examined the serotonin 1A receptor polymorphism (5-HTR1A). Koreans and European Americans were genotyped and reported their chronic locus of attention. They found a significant interaction between 5-HTR1A and culture in the locus of attention. Koreans reported attending to the field more than European Americans, and this cultural difference was moderated by 5-HTR1A. There was a linear pattern such that those homozygous for the G allele, which is associated with reduced ability to adapt to changes in reinforcement, more strongly endorsed the culturally reinforced mode of thinking than those homozygous for the C allele, with those heterozygous in the middle. Kim *et al.* claim that their findings suggest that the same genetic predisposition can result in divergent psychological outcomes, depending on an individual's cultural context.

The sample used in this study included 149 Korean and 140 European subjects. Given the problems with the Caspi *et al.* work, it is clear that replication across larger samples will be needed.

That being said, the results of H. Kim *et al.* do indeed underline the necessity of expanding work on psychiatric disorders to gene-culture-environment interactions. It seems likely, however, that, overall, culture-environment interaction effects will predominate.

5.3   Global Broadcast Models

Recent research on schizophrenia, dyslexia, and autism broadly supports a 'brain connectivity' perspective on these disorders of considerable interest from the viewpoint of global broadcast models.

For example, Burns *et al.* (2003), on the basis of sophisticated diffusion tensor magnetic resonance imaging studies, argue that schizophrenia is a disorder of large-scale neurocognitive networks rather than specific regions, and that pathological changes in the disorder should be sought at the supra-regional level. Both structural and functional abnormalities in frontoparietal networks have been described and may constitute a basis for the wide range of cognitive functions impaired in the disorder, such as selective attention, language processing and attribution of agency.

Silani *et al.* (2005) find that, for dyslexia, altered activation observed within the reading system is associated with altered density of grey and white matter of specific brain regions, such as the left middle and inferior temporal gyri and left arcuate fasciculus. This supports the view that dyslexia is associated with both local grey matter dysfunction and with altered larger scale connectivity among phonological/reading areas.

Villalobos *et al.* (2005) explore the hypothesis that large-scale abnormalities of the dorsal stream and possibly the mirror neuron system, may be responsible for impairments of joint attention, imitation, and secondarily for language delays in autism. Their empirical study showed that those with autism had significantly reduced connectivity with bilateral inferior frontal area 44, which is compatible with the hypothesis of mirror neuron defects in autism. More generally, their results suggest that dorsal stream connectivity in autism may not be fully functional.

Courchesne and Pierce (2005) suggest that, for autism, connectivity within the frontal lobe is excessive, disorganized, and inadequately selective, whereas connectivity between frontal cortex and other systems is poorly synchronized, weakly responsive and information impoverished. Increased local but reduced long-distance cortical–cortical reciprocal activity and coupling would impair the fundamental frontal function of integrating information from widespread and diverse systems and providing complex context-rich feedback, guidance and control to lower-level systems.

Coplan (2005) has observed a striking pattern of excessive frontal lobe self-connectivity in certain cases of anxiety disorder, and Coplan *et al.* (2005) find that maternal stress can affect long-term hippocampal neurodevelopment in a primate model.

As stated, brain connectivity is the *sine qua non* of global broadcast models of consciousness, and further analysis suggests that these disorders cannot be fully understood in the absence of a functional theory of consciousness, and in particular, of a detailed understanding of the elaborate regulatory mechanisms which must have evolved over the past half billion years to ensure the stability of that most central and most powerful of adaptations. For humans, of course, one of the principal regulatory mechanisms for mental function is the embedding culture and culturally mediated social interaction, in addition to culture's role as the second system of human heritage. As the evolutionary anthropologist Robert Boyd has put it, culture is as much a part of human biology as the enamel on our teeth (Richerson and Boyd, 2006).

Distortion of consciousness is not simply an epiphenomenon of the emotional dysregulation many see as the 'real' cause of mental disorder. Like the pervasive effects of culture, distortion of consciousness lies at the heart of both the individual experience of mental disorder and the effect of it on the embedding of the individual within both social relationships and cultural or environmental context. Yet the experience of individual consciousness cannot be disentangled from social interaction and culture (Wallace, 2005). Distortion of a culturally mediated consciousness in mental disorders inhibits both routine social interchange and the ability to meet internalized or expected cultural norms, a potentially destabilizing positive feedback. Distortion of consciousness profoundly affects the ability to learn new, or change old, skills in the face of changing patterns of threat or opportunity, perhaps the most critical purpose of the adaptation itself. Distortion of consciousness causing decoupling from social and cultural context is usually a threat to long-term individual survival, and those with mental disorders significantly affecting consciousness typically experience severely shortened lifespans.

Recent exploration of a cognitive paradigm for gene expression (Wallace and Wallace, 2008, 2009) incorporates the effects of surrounding epigenetic regulatory machinery as a kind of catalyst to include the effects of the embedding information source of human culture on the ontology of the human mind. The essential feature, as argued above at great length, is that a cognitive process, including gene expression, can instantiate a dual information source that can interact with the generalized language of culture in which, for example, social interplay and the interpretation of socioeconomic and environmental stressors, involve complicated matters of symbolism and its grammar and syntax. These information sources interact by a crosstalk that, over the life course, profoundly influences the ontology of mind, including its manifold dysfunctions.

That is, contemporary American work on gene–environment interactions in psychiatry must be extended to the study of gene–culture–environment interactions.

5.4   Gene Expression

To recapitulate somewhat the arguments of Section 4.4, a cognitive paradigm for gene expression has emerged in which contextual factors determine the behavior of what Cohen characterizes as a 'reactive system', not at all a deterministic, or even stochastic, mechanical process (e.g., Cohen, 2006; Cohen and Harel, 2007; Wallace and Wallace, 2008, 2009). The very different formal approaches are, however, all in the spirit of Maturana and Varela (1980, 1992) who understood the central role that cognitive process must play across a vast array of biological phenomena.

O'Nuallain (2008) has placed gene expression firmly in the realm of complex linguistic behavior, for which context imposes meaning, claiming that the analogy between gene expression and language production is useful both as a fruitful research paradigm and also, given the relative lack of success of natural language processing by computer, as a cautionary tale for molecular biology.

A relatively simple model of cognitive process as an information source permits use of Dretske's (1994) insight that any cognitive phenomenon must be constrained by the limit theorems of information theory, in the same sense that sums of stochastic variables are constrained by the central limit theorem.

This perspective permits a new formal approach to gene expression and its dysfunctions, in particular suggesting new and powerful statistical tools for data analysis that could contribute to exploring both ontology and its pathologies. Wallace and Wallace (2009, 2010) apply the perspective, respectively, to infectious and chronic disease. It is easy to extend the mathematical foundations of that work to include the context of an embedding information source representing the compelling varieties of human culture.

This approach is consistent with the broad context of epigenetics and epigenetic epidemiology. In particular, Jablonka and Lamb (1995, 1998) argue that information can be transmitted from one generation to the next in ways other than through the base sequence of DNA. It can be transmitted through cultural and behavioral means in higher animals, and by epigenetic means in cell lineages. All of these transmission systems allow the inheritance of environmentally induced variation. Such Epigenetic Inheritance Systems are the memory systems that enable somatic cells of different phenotypes but identical genotypes to transmit their phenotypes to their descendants, even when the stimuli that originally induced these phenotypes are no longer present.

After a decade of research and debate, the epigenetic perspective has received much empirical confirmation (e.g., Backdahl *et al.* 2009; Turner, 2000; Jaenisch and Bird, 2003; Jablonka, 2004).

Foley *et al.* (2009) argue that epimutation is estimated to be a hundred times more frequent than genetic mutation and may occur randomly or in response to the environment. Periods of rapid cell division and epigenetic remodeling are likely to be most sensitive to stochastic or environmentally mediated epimutation. Disruption of epigenetic profile is a feature of most cancers and is speculated to play a role in the etiology of other complex diseases including asthma allergy, obesity, type 2 diabetes, coronary heart disease, autism spectrum disorders, bipolar disorders and schizophrenia.

Scherrer and Jost (2007a, b) explicitly invoke information theory in their extension of the definition of the gene to include the local epigenetic machinery, a construct they term the 'genon'. Their central point is that coding information is not simply contained in the coded sequence, but is, in their terms, *provided by* the genon that accompanies it on the expression pathway and controls in which peptide it will end up. In their view, the information that counts is not about the identity of a nucleotide or an amino acid derived from it, but about the relative frequency of the transcription and generation of a particular type of coding sequence that then contributes to the determination of the types and numbers of functional products derived from the DNA coding region under consideration.

The proper formal tools for understanding phenomena that 'provide' information – that are information sources – are the rate distortion theorem and its zero error limit, the Shannon–McMillan theorem.

5.5   Summary

Culturally structured psychosocial stress, and similar noxious exposures, can write distorted images of themselves onto human ontology – both child growth, and, if sufficiently powerful, adult development as well – by a variety of mechanisms, initiating a punctuated trajectory to characteristic forms of comorbid mind/body dysfunction. Following the arguments of Chapters 3 and 4, this occurs in a manner recognizably analogous to resilience domain shifts affecting stressed ecosystems (e.g., Wallace, 2008; Holling, 1973; Gunderson, 2000). Consequently, like ecosystem restoration, reversal or palliation may often be exceedingly difficult once a generalized domain shift has taken place. Thus a public health approach to the prevention of mental disorders may be paramount: rather than seeking to understand why half a population does not respond to the LD50 of a teratogenic environmental exposure, one seeks policies and social reforms that limit the exposure.

Both socio-cultural and epigenetic environmental influences – like gene methylation – are heritable, in addition to genetic mechanisms. The missing heritability of complex diseases that Manolio *et al.* (2009) seek to find in more and better gene studies is most likely dispersed within the 'dark matter' of these two other systems of heritage that together constitute the larger, and likely synergistic – and cognitive – regulatory machinery for gene expression. More and more purely genetic studies would, under such circumstances, be akin to using increasingly powerful microscopes to look for cosmic membranes of strewn galaxies.

A crucial matter is the conversion of the probability models we proposed in Chapters 1–3 into statistical tools suitable for analyzing real data. The difficulty involves not just programming such models for use, but identifying appropriate real-world problems, assembling available data sets, transforming the data as needed for the models, and actually applying the statistical models. Indeed, the environmental health literature contains numerous examples of developmental deviations due to either chemical exposures or interaction between chemical and socioeconomic exposures, and these could serve as sources of data for direct analysis (e.g., Needleman *et al.*, 1996;

Fullilove, 2004; Dietrich *et al.*, 2001; Miranda *et al.*, 2007; Glass *et al.*, 2009; Jacobson and Jacobson, 2003; Shankardass *et al.*, 2009; Clougherty *et al.*, 2007; Ben Jonathan *et al.*, 2009; Karp *et al.*, 2005; Sarlio-Lahteenkorva and Lahelma, 2001; Wallace and Wallace, 2005; Wallace, Wallace and Rauh, 2003). Thus, quite a number of data sets exist in the environmental health and socioeconomic epidemiological literature that could be subjected to meta-analysis and other review for model verification and fitting. The probability models invoked here, when converted to statistical tools for data analysis, hold great potential for understanding developmental trajectories and interfering factors (teratogens) through the life course. Sets of crosscultural variants of these data focusing specifically on mental disorders, would be needed to address the particular concerns of this chapter.

Nonetheless, the general approach of this work is of no small interest for understanding the ontology of the human mind and its pathologies. West-Eberhard (2003, 2005) argues that any new input, whether it comes from the genome, like a mutation, or from the external environment, like a temperature change, a pathogen, or a parental opinion, has a developmental effect only if the preexisting phenotype is responsive to it. A new input causes a reorganization of the phenotype, or 'developmental recombination'. In developmental recombination, phenotypic traits are expressed in new or distinctive combinations during ontogeny, or undergo correlated quantitative change in dimensions. Developmental recombination can result in evolutionary divergence at all levels of organization.

According to West-Eberhard, individual development can be visualized as a series of branching pathways. Each branch point is a developmental decision, or switch point, governed by some regulatory apparatus, and each switch point defines a modular trait. Developmental recombination implies the origin or deletion of a branch and a new or lost modular trait. The novel regulatory response and the novel trait originate simultaneously. Their origins are, in fact, inseparable events: there cannot, West-Eberhard concludes, be a change in the phenotype, a novel phenotypic state, without an altered developmental pathway.

The nested, multilevel, cognitive paradigm analyses of the previous chapters provide a new formal picture of this process: the normal branching of developmental trajectories, and the disruptive impacts of teratogenic events of various kinds, can be described in terms of a growing sequence of dual information sources representing patterns of cognitive gene expression catalyzed by epigenetic information sources that, for humans, must include culture and culturally modulated social interaction as well as more direct mechanisms like gene methylation. This is a novel way of looking at human development and its disorders that may prove to be of some use. The most important innovation of this work, however, seems to be the natural incorporation of the external information source of embedding culture as an essential component of the epigenetic regulation of human development, and in the effects of environment on the expression of mental disorders, bringing what is perhaps the central reality of human biology into the center of contemporary biological psychiatry.

In sum, we have outlined a broad class of nested cognition probability models of gene–culture–environment interaction, and suggested some statistical tools based on them, that might help current studies of gene–environment interaction in American psychiatry avoid Heine's (2001) trap of developing an understanding of the self, and its disorders, that is peculiar in the context of the world's cultures.

Chapter 6

EXAMPLE: PROTEIN FOLDING

6.1 Introduction

The existence of 'global' protein folding and aggregation diseases, in conjunction with the elaborate cellular folding regulatory apparatus associated with the endoplasmic reticulum and other structures (e.g., Scheuner and Kaufman, 2008; Dobson, 2003) makes clear that simple physical 'folding funnel' free energy mechanisms are not fully adequate to describe the process, in spite of the fundamental observation of Anfinsen (1973) that denatured proteins refold in aqueous solution at low concentrations. This suggests that, for *in vivo* conditions, a more biologically based model is needed, analogous to Atlan and Cohen's (1998) cognitive paradigm for the immune system. That is, the intractable set of disorders related to protein aggregation and misfolding belies simple mechanistic approaches, although free energy landscape pictures surely capture part of the process. The diseases range from prion illnesses like Creutzfeld–Jakob disease, to amyloid-related dysfunctions like Alzheimer's, Huntington's, and Parkinson's diseases, and type 2 diabetes. Misfolding disorders include emphysema and cystic fibrosis. A deeper understanding of protein folding mechanisms, in particular of epigenetic, social, and environmental influences, might contribute to prevention and treatment of these debilitating conditions.

Indeed, the role of epigenetic and environmental factors in type 2 diabetes has long been known (e.g., Zhang *et al.*, 2009; Wallach and Rey, 2009). Haataja *et al.* (2008), for example, conclude that the islet in type 2 diabetes shows much in common with neuropathology in neurodegenerative diseases where interest is now focused on protein misfolding and aggregation and the diseases are now often referred to as unfolded protein diseases.

Scheuner and Kaufman (2008) likewise examine the unfolded protein response in β cell failure and diabetes. Their opening paragraph raises fundamental questions regarding the adequacy of simple energy landscape models of protein folding:

> In eukaryotic cells, protein synthesis and secretion are precisely coupled with the capacity of the endoplasmic reticulum (ER) to fold, process, and traffic proteins to the cell surface. These processes are coupled through several signal transduction pathways collectively known as the unfolded protein response [that] functions to reduce the amount of nascent protein that enters the ER lumen, to increase the ER capacity to fold protein through transcriptional up-regulation of ER chaperones and folding catalysts, and to induce degradation of misfolded and aggregated protein.

Qiu *et al.* (2009), on a quite different scale, address Alzheimer's disease in much the same fashion:

> Alzheimer's dementia is a multifactorial disease in which older age is the strongest risk factor... [that] may partially reflect the cumulative effects of different risk and protective factors over the lifespan, including the complex interactions of genetic susceptibility, psychosocial factors, biological factors, and environmental exposures experienced over the lifespan.

Qiu *et al.* (2009) explain that mutation effects account for only a small fraction of observed cases, and that the APOE ϵ4 allele – the only established genetic factor for both early and late onset disease – is a *susceptibility* gene, neither necessary nor sufficient for disease onset. They further describe how many of the same factors implicated in diabetes and cardiovascular disease predict onset of Alzheimer's as well: tobacco use, high blood pressure, high serum cholesterol, chronic inflammation, as indexed by a higher level of serum C-reactive protein, and diabetes itself. Significant protective factors include high educational and socioeconomic status, regular physical exercise, mentally demanding activities, and extensive social engagement.

Similarly, Fillit *et al.* (2008) find that lifestyle risk factors for cardiovascular disease, such as obesity, lack of exercise, smoking, and certain psychosocial factors, have been associated with an increased risk for cognitive decline and dementia, concluding that current evidence indicates an association with hypertension, dyslipidemia, and diabetes.

Goldschmidt *et al.* (2010) describe pathological protein fibrillation as follows:

We found that [protein segments with high fibrillation propensity] tend to be buried or twisted into unfavorable conformations for forming beta sheets... For some proteins a delicate balance between protein folding and misfolding exists that can be tipped by changes in environment, destabilizing mutations, or even protein concentration...

In addition to the self-chaperoning effects described above, proteins are also protected from fibrillation during the process of folding by molecular chaperones...

Our genome-wide analysis revealed that self-complementary segments are found in almost all proteins, yet not all proteins are amyloids. The implication is that chaperoning effects have evolved to constrain self-complementary segments from interaction with each other.

These processes and mechanisms seem no less examples of chemical cognition than the immune/inflammatory responses that Atlan and Cohen (1998) describe in terms of an explicit cognitive paradigm, or that characterizes well-studied neural processes. Our own work (Wallace and Wallace, 2008, 2009) introduces a similar, and highly formal, cognitive paradigm for gene expression whose machinery permits the natural incorporation of epigenetic and environmental signals via catalytic mechanisms similar to those of Section 2.3 above. The implication is that progress in understanding, preventing, and treating protein folding and aggregation disorders now requires introduction of a biologically based cognitive paradigm for the folding process itself.

The symmetries and dynamics of protein folding are striking and, in a local sense, fairly well understood (Dill *et al.* 2007; Wolynes, 1996; Onuchic and Wolynes, 2004). Goodsell and Olson (2000) show several typical examples. More general, but less overtly 'symmetric' conformations, however, involve finite tilings of helices, sheets, and attachment loops that would seem better described using groupoid methods, following the arguments of Weinstein (1996): as Wolynes (1996) put the matter, "It is the inexact symmetries of biological molecules that are most striking".

Anfinsen's (1973) thermodynamic hypothesis has strongly dominated thinking on the subject: the native state of a protein has the lowest Gibbs free energy, determined by the interaction of the amino acid sequence and the embedding environment (Wolynes, 1996), with hydrophobic amino acids driven into the center of the 'native' folded protein structure. More recent work (e.g., summarized in Lei and Huang, 2010) suggests that large, complex proteins may have native configurations representing kinetically accessible, rather than thermodynamically minimal, states. Andre *et al.* (2008) explore the central insight that "...selection is only likely to operate on primordial complexes with sufficient initial interaction energy to at least partially overcome the entropic costs of association of the monomers; evolution can only optimize a complex that is populated sufficiently to confer a benefit on the organism".

It seems possible to finesse this general perspective by invoking a rate distortion argument applied to the transmitted signal represented by the translation of the genome into the final, evolutionarily driven, condensation of the molten globule of the resulting amino acid string. The argument, an adaptation of Tlusty's (2007) insights regarding the role of rate distortion constraints in evolutionary process, seems fairly direct. It is based on standard material from statistical physics and information theory, using, respectively, average distortion and the rate distortion function itself, as temperature analogs to produce mirror image 'energy' and 'development' pictures of protein folding.

The final step is to mathematically 'weaken', i.e., generalize, the development perspective, using information sources formally dual to the several chemical cognitive processes involved in protein folding. These then, in a sense, engage in a local, multifactorial, coevolutionary interaction whose quasi-stable dynamic states generate products that are, respectively, correct, repaired, eliminated, or misfolded/aggregated proteins. This set of processes is analogous to quasi-stable ecosystem resilience modes, in the sense of Holling (1973) or Gunderson (2000), and apparently subject to punctuated transitions between them consequent on epigenetic or environmental perturbations. The formalism is a version of that presented in Chapter 3.

The argument generates a new class of statistical models based on the asymptotic limit theorems of information, in the same sense that regression and other parametric models are based on the central limit theorem, and these should prove useful in data analysis as well as providing a new conceptual approach.

We begin with a restatement of some standard material from statistical physics that provides the basis for a subsequent argument-by-abduction.

6.2 Spontaneous Symmetry Breaking

Landau's theory of phase transitions (Landau and Lifshitz, 2007) assumes that the free energy of a system near criticality can be expanded in a power series of some 'order parameter' ϕ representing a fundamental measurable quantity, that is, a symmetry invariant. One writes

$$F_0 = \sum_{k=m}^{p(>m)} A_k \phi^k \,, \tag{6.1}$$

with $A_2 \approx \alpha(T - T_c)$ sufficiently close to the critical temperature T_c. This mean field approach can be used to describe a variety of second-order effects for $p = 4$ or $p = 6$, $A_3 = 0$ and $A_4 > 0$, and first order phase transitions (requiring latent heat) for either $p = 6, A_3 = 0, A_4 < 0$ or $p = 4$ and $A_3 \neq 0$. These can be both temperature induced (for $m = 2$) and field induced (for $m = 1$).

Minimization of F_0 with respect to the order parameter yields the average value of ϕ, $< \phi >$, which is zero above the critical temperature and non-zero below it. In the absence of external fields, the second-order transition occurs at $T = T_c$, while the first-order, needing latent heat, occurs at $T_c^* = T_c + A_4^2/4\alpha A_6$. In the latter case thermal hysteresis arises between $T_s \equiv T_c + A_4^2/3\alpha A_6$ and T_c. A more accurate approximation involves an expression that recognizes the effect of coarse-graining, adding a term in $\nabla^2 \phi$ and integrating over space rather than summing. Regimes dominated by this gradient will show behaviors analogous to those described using the one-dimensional Landau–Ginzburg equation, which, among other things, characterizes superconductivity.

The Landau formalism quickly enters deep topological waters (Pettini, 2007, pp. 42–43; Landau and Lifshitz, 2007, pp. 459–466), to recall something of the arguments of Chapter 3, the essence of Landau's insight was that phase transitions without latent heat – second order transitions – were usually in the context of a significant symmetry change in the physical states of a system, with one phase, at higher temperature, being far more symmetric than the other. A symmetry is lost in the transition, a phenomenon called spontaneous symmetry breaking. The greatest possible set of symmetries in a physical system is that of the Hamiltonian describing its energy states. Usually states accessible at lower temperatures will lack symmetries available at higher temperatures, so that the lower temperature phase is the less symmetric: the randomization of higher temperatures ensures that higher symmetry/energy states will then be accessible to the system.

This can be formalized, following Pettini (2007), as follows. Consider a thermodynamic system having a free energy F which is a function of temperature T, pressure P, and some other extensive macroscopic parameters m_i, so that $F = F(P, T, m_i)$. The m_i all vanish in the most symmetric phase, so that, as a function of the m_i, $F(P, T, m_i)$ is invariant with respect to the transformations of the symmetry group G_0 of the most symmetric phase of the system when all $m_i \equiv 0$.

The state of the system can be represented by a vector $|m >= |m_1, ..., m_n >$ in a vector space $\mathcal{E}$. Now, within $\mathcal{E}$, construct a linear representation of the group G_0 that associates with any $g \in G_0$ a matrix $M(g)$ having rank n. In general, the representation $M(g)$ is reducible, and we can decompose $\mathcal{E}$ into invariant irreducible subspaces $\mathcal{E}_1, \mathcal{E}_2, ..., \mathcal{E}_k$, having basis vectors $|e_i^{(n)} >$ with $n = 1, 2, ...n_i$ and $n_i = dim\mathcal{E}_i$. The state variables m_i are transformed into new variables $\eta_i^{(n)} =< e_i^{(n)} | m >$, where the bracket represents an inner product.

In terms of irreducible representations $D_i(g)$ induced by $M(g)$ in $\mathcal{E}_i$,

$$M(g) = D_1(g) \oplus D_2(g) \oplus, ..., \oplus D_k(g).$$

If at least one of the $\eta_i^{(n)}$ is nonzero, then the system no longer has the symmetry G_0. This symmetry has been broken, and the new symmetry group is G_i, associated with the representation $D_i(g)$ in $\mathcal{E}_i$. The variables $\eta_i^{(n)}$ are the new order parameters, and the free energy is now $F = F(P, T, \eta_i^{(n)})$. For a physical system the actual values of the η as functions of P and T can be variationally determined by minimizing the free energy F.

Two essential features distinguish information systems, like the translation of a genome into a folded protein, from this simple physical model.

First, the dynamics of order parameters cannot always be determined by simplistic minimization procedures in biological circumstances (e.g., Levinthal, 1969): embedding environments can, within contextual constraints (that particularly include available metabolic free energy), write images of themselves via evolutionary selection mechanisms, driving the system toward such structures as the protein folding funnel (e.g., Levinthal, 1968; Wolynes, 1996).

Second, the essential symmetry of information sources is quite often driven by groupoid, rather than group, structures (e.g., Wallace, 2010). One must then engage the full transitive orbit/isotropy group decomposition, and examine groupoid representations (Bos, 2007; Buneci, 2003) configured about the irreducible representations of the isotropy groups. This observation seems particularly relevant given the usual helix/sheet/connecting loop tilings that characterize most elaborate protein conformations (Wolynes, 1996).

A brief summary of standard material on groupoids is included as a Mathematical Appendix.

6.3   A Formal Approach

Here we think of the machinery listing a sequence of codons as communicating with machinery that produces amino acids, folds them *in context*, and produces the final symmetric protein. Suppose it possible to compare what is actually produced with what should have been produced, perhaps by a simple evolutionary survival mechanism, perhaps via some more sophisticated error-correcting systems. This is not a new idea, and Onuchic and Wolynes (2004), for example, put the matter fully in evolutionary terms:

> Protein folding should be complex...a folding mechanism must involve a complex network of elementary interactions. However, simple empirical patterns of protein folding kinetics...have been shown to exist.

> This simplicity is owed to the global organization of the landscape of the energies of protein conformations into a funnel... This organization is not characteristic of all polymers with any sequence of amino acids, but is a result of evolution...

> Evolution achieves robustness by selecting for sequences in which the interactions present in the functionally useful structure are not in conflict, as in a random heteropolymer, but instead are mutually supportive and cooperatively lead to a low energy structure. The interactions are 'minimally frustrated'...or 'consistent'...

It is possible to reframe something of this mechanism in explicit information theory terms, and invoke the rate distortion theorem, recapitulating the argument in terms of protein folding dynamics.

Suppose a sequence of signals is generated by a biological information source Y having output $y^n = y_1, y_2, ...$ – codons. This is 'digitized' in terms of the observed behavior of the system with which it communicates, say a sequence of 'observed behaviors' $b^n = b_1, b_2, ...$ – here, amino acids and their folded protein structure. Assume each b^n is then deterministically retranslated back into a reproduction of the original biological signal,

$b^n \rightarrow \hat{y}^n = \hat{y}_1, \hat{y}_2, ...$

Define a distortion measure $d(y, \hat{y})$ comparing the original to the retranslated path. As described in the Mathematical Appendix, many distortion measures are possible.

The distortion between *paths* y^n and $\hat{y}^n$ is defined as

$$d(y^n, \hat{y}^n) \equiv \frac{1}{n} \sum_{j=1}^{n} d(y_j, \hat{y}_j).$$

A remarkable fact of the rate distortion theorem is that *the basic result is independent of the exact distortion measure chosen* (Cover and Thomas, 2006; Dembo and Zeitouni, 1998).

Suppose that with each path y^n and b^n-path retranslation into the y-language, denoted $\hat{y}^n$, there are associated individual, joint, and conditional probability distributions $p(y^n), p(\hat{y}^n), p(y^n, \hat{y}^n), p(y^n|\hat{y}^n)$.

Again, the average distortion is

$$D \equiv \sum_{y^n} p(y^n) d(y^n, \hat{y}^n).$$

The information transmitted from the Y to the $\hat{Y}$ process is

$$I(Y, \hat{Y}) \equiv H(Y) - H(Y|\hat{Y}) = H(Y) + H(\hat{Y}) - H(Y, \hat{Y}),$$

where $H(..., ...)$ is the joint, and $H(...|...)$ the conditional, Shannon uncertainties (Cover and Thomas, 2006; Ash, 1990).

Recall that if there is no uncertainty in Y given the retranslation $\hat{Y}$, then no information is lost, and the systems are in perfect synchrony. In general, of course, this will not be true.

Again, the *rate distortion function* $R(D)$ for a source Y with a distortion measure $d(y, \hat{y})$ is

$$R(D) = \min_{p(y,\hat{y}); \sum_{(y,\hat{y})} p(y)p(y|\hat{y})d(y,\hat{y}) \leq D} I(Y, \hat{Y}).$$

The minimization is over all conditional distributions $p(y|\hat{y})$ for which the joint distribution $p(y, \hat{y}) = p(y)p(y|\hat{y})$ satisfies the average distortion constraint (i.e., average distortion $\leq D$).

To reiterate, the *rate distortion theorem* states that $R(D)$ is the minimum necessary rate of information transmission which ensures the communication between the biological vesicles does not exceed average distortion D. Thus, $R(D)$ defines a minimum necessary channel capacity. Cover and Thomas (2006) or Dembo and Zeitouni (1998) provide details.

Again, an absolutely central fact characterizing the rate distortion function: Cover and Thomas (2006) show that $R(D)$ *is necessarily a decreasing convex function of D for any reasonable definition of distortion.*

That is, $R(D)$ *is always* a reverse J-shaped curve. This will prove crucial for the overall argument. Indeed, convexity is an exceedingly powerful mathematical condition, and permits deep inference (e.g., Rockafellar, 1970). Ellis (1985, Ch. VI) applies convexity theory to conventional statistical mechanics.

Recall, again, the relation between information source uncertainty and channel capacity (e.g., Ash, 1990), $H[X] \leq C$, where H is the uncertainty of the source X. C is the the channel capacity, defined according to the relation (Ash, 1990) $C \equiv \max_{P(X)} I(X|Y)$ where $P(X)$ is chosen so as to maximize the rate of information transmission along a channel Y.

Recall from Chapter 3 the homology between information source uncertainty and free energy density.

Conversely, information source uncertainty has an important heuristic interpretation that Ash (1990) describes as follows:

> [W]e may regard a portion of text in a particular language as being produced by an information source. The probabilities $P[X_n = a_n | X_0 = a_0, ... X_{n-1} = a_{n-1}]$ may be estimated from the available data about the language; in this way we can estimate the uncertainty associated with the language. A large uncertainty means, by the [Shannon–McMillan theorem], a large number of 'meaningful' sequences. Thus given two languages with uncertainties H_1 and H_2 respectively, if $H_1 > H_2$, then in the absence of noise it is easier to communicate in the first language; more can be said in the same amount of time. On the other hand, it will be easier to reconstruct a scrambled portion of text in the second language, since fewer of the possible sequences of length n are meaningful.

In sum, if a biological system characterized by H_1 has a richer and more complicated internal communication structure than one characterized by H_2, then necessarily $H_1 > H_2$ and system 1 represents a more energetic process than system 2, and by the arguments of Section 2.3 and Eq. (3.4), may trigger even greater metabolic free energy dynamics, as is shown in more detail in Chapter 3.

As described in Chapter 3, the rate distortion function, $R(D)$ is also a free energy measure, constrained by the availability of metabolic free energy.

6.4   The Energy Picture

Ash's comment leads directly to a model in which the average distortion between the initial codon stream and the final form of the folded amino acid stream, the protein, becomes a dominant force, particularly in an evolutionary context in which fidelity of codon expression has survival value. The direct model examines the distortion between the codon stream and the folded protein structure.

Suppose there are n possible folding schemes. The most familiar approach, perhaps, is to assume that a given distortion measure, D, under evolutionary selection constraints, serves much as an external temperature bath for the possible distribution of conformation free energies, the set $\{\mathcal{H}_1, ..., \mathcal{H}_n\}$. That is, high distortion, represented by a low rate of transmission of information between codon machine and amino acid/protein folding machine, permits a larger distribution of possible symmetries – the big end of the folding funnel – according to the classic formula

$$Pr[\mathcal{H}_j] = \frac{\exp[-\mathcal{H}_j/\lambda D]}{\sum_{i=1}^{n} \exp[-\mathcal{H}_i/\lambda D]}, \qquad (6.2)$$

where $Pr[\mathcal{H}_j]$ is the probability of folding scheme j having conformational free energy $\mathcal{H}_j$.

$Pr[\mathcal{H}_j]$ is a one parameter distribution in the 'intensive' quantity D. The free energy Morse function associated with this probability is

$$F_R = -\lambda D \log[\sum_{i=1}^{n} \exp[-\mathcal{H}_i/\lambda D]]. \qquad (6.3)$$

Applying a spontaneous symmetry breaking argument to F_R generates topological transitions in folded protein structure as the 'temperature' D decreases, i.e., as the average distortion declines. That is, as the channel capacity connecting codon machines with amino acid/protein folding machines increases, the system is driven to a particular conformation, according to the 'protein folding funnel'.

See the Mathematical Appendix for an outline of Morse theory.

6.5   The Developmental Picture

The developmental approach of Wallace and Wallace (2009) permits a different perspective on protein folding. The central concern is developmental pathways in a 'phenotype space' that, in a series of steps, take the amino acid string $\mathbf{S}_0$ at time 0 to the final folded conformation $\mathbf{S}_f$ at some time t in a long series of distinct, sequential, intermediate configurations $\mathbf{S}_i$.

Let $N(n)$ be the number of possible paths of length n that lead from $\mathbf{S}_0$ to $\mathbf{S}_f$. The essential assumptions are:

1. This is a highly systematic process governed by a 'grammar' and 'syntax' driven by the folding funnel, so that it is possible to divide all possible paths $x_n = \{\mathbf{S}_0, \mathbf{S}_1, ..., \mathbf{S}_n\}$ into two sets, a small, high probability subset that conforms to the demands of the folding funnel topology, and a much larger 'nonsense' subset having vanishingly small probability.

2. If $N(n)$ is the number of high probability paths of length n, then the 'ergodic' limit $H = \lim_{n\to\infty} \log[N(n)]/n$ both exists and is independent of the path x. This is, essentially, a restatement of the Shannon–McMillan theorem (Khinchin, 1957).

That is, the folding of a particular protein, from its amino acid string to its final form, is not a random event, but represents a highly – evolutionarily – structured (i.e., by the folding funnel) 'statement' by an information source having source uncertainty H.

Symmetry arguments

A formal equivalence class algebra can now be constructed by choosing different origin and end points $\mathbf{S}_0, \mathbf{S}_f$ and defining equivalence of two states by the existence of a high-probability meaningful path connecting them with the same origin and end. Disjoint partition by equivalence class, analogous to orbit equivalence classes for dynamical systems, defines the vertices of the proposed network of developmental protein 'languages'. We thus envision a *network of metanetworks*. Each vertex then represents a different equivalence class of developmental information sources. This is an abstract set of metanetwork 'languages'.

This structure generates a groupoid, in the sense of Weinstein (1996). States a_j, a_k in a set A are related by the groupoid morphism if and only if there exists a high-probability grammatical path connecting them to the same base and end points, and tuning across the various possible ways in which that can happen – the different developmental languages – parameterizes the set of equivalence relations and creates the (very large) groupoid.

There is an implicit hierarchy. First, there is structure *within the system having the same base and end points*. Second, there is a complicated groupoid structure defined by sets of dual information sources surrounding the variation of base and end points. It is not necessary to know what that structure is in any detail, but its existence has profound implications.

The first step is to start with the simplest case, the set of dual information sources associated with a fixed pair of beginning and end states.

The first level

Taking the serial grammar/syntax model above, not all high probability meaningful paths from S_0 to S_f are actually the same. They are structured by the uncertainty of the associated dual information source, and that has a homological relation with free energy density.

Index possible information sources connecting base and end points by some set $A = \cup \alpha$. Argument by abduction from statistical physics is direct. The minimum channel capacity needed to produce average distortion less than D in the energy picture above is $R(D)$. Take the probability of a particular H_β as determined by the standard expression

$$P[H_\beta] = \frac{\exp[-H_\beta/\mu R]}{\sum_\alpha \exp[-H_\alpha/\mu R]} \,, \tag{6.4}$$

where the sum may, in fact, be a complicated abstract integral. A basic requirement, then, is that the sum/integral always converges.

Thus, in this formulation, there must be structure *within* a (cross sectional) connected component in the base configuration space, determined by R. Some dual information sources will be 'richer'/smarter than others, but, conversely, must use more available channel capacity for their completion.

The second level

While it is possible to simply impose an equivalence class structure based on equal levels of energy/source uncertainty, producing a groupoid (and possibly allowing a Morse theory approach), the argument can be generalized *by now allowing both source and end points to vary*, as well as by imposing energy-level equivalence. This produces a far more highly structured groupoid.

Equivalence classes define groupoids by standard mechanisms. The basic equivalence classes – here involving both information source uncertainty level and the variation of S_0 and S_f, will define transitive groupoids, and higher order systems can be constructed by the union of transitive groupoids, having larger alphabets that allow more complicated statements in the sense of Ash (1990) above.

Again, given a minimum necessary channel capacity R, the metabolic-energy-constrained probability of an information source representing equivalence class G_i, H_{G_i}, will be given by

$$P[H_{G_i}] = \frac{\exp[-H_{G_i}/\kappa R]}{\sum_j \exp[-H_{G_j}/\kappa R]} \,, \tag{6.5}$$

where the sum/integral is over all possible elements of the largest available symmetry groupoid. By the arguments of Ash (1990) above, compound sources, formed by the union of underlying transitive groupoids, being more complex, generally having richer alphabets, as it were, will all have higher free-energy-density-equivalents than those of the base (transitive) groupoids.

Let

$$Z_G = \sum_j \exp[-H_{G_j}/\kappa R]. \tag{6.6}$$

Define the *groupoid free energy* of the system, a Morse function F_G, at channel capacity R, as

$$F_G[R] = -\kappa R \log[Z_G[R]]. \tag{6.7}$$

These free energy constructs permit introduction of the spontaneous symmetry breaking arguments above, but now an *increase* in R (with corresponding decrease in average distortion D) permits richer system dynamics – higher source uncertainty – resulting in more rapid transmission of the 'message' constituting convergence from S_0 to S_f.

Again, see the Mathematical Appendix for a summary of Morse theory results.

Folding speed and mechanism

Dill *et al.* (2007) describe the conundrum of folding speeds as follows:

...[P]rotein folding speeds – now known to vary over more than eight orders of magnitude – correlate with the topology of the native protein: fast folders usually have mostly local structure, such as helices and tight turns, whereas slow folders usually have more non-local structure, such as β sheets (Plaxco *et al.*, 1998)...

A simple groupoid probability argument reproduces this result. Assume that protein structure can be characterized by some groupoid representing, at least, the disjoint union of the groups describing the symmetries of component secondary structures – helices and sheets. Then, in Eq. (6.5), the set $A = \cup\alpha$ grows in size – cardinality – with increasing structural complexity. If channel capacity is capped by some mechanism, so that (at least) R grows at a lesser rate than A, by some measure, then

$$P[H_\beta] = \frac{\exp[-H_\beta/\mu R]}{\sum_\alpha \exp[-H_\alpha/\mu R]}$$

must decrease with increase in the number of possible states α, i.e., with increase in the cardinality of A, producing progressively lower rates of convergence to the final state. Wallace (2010a) provides more details.

These matters lead to the next central question: how can folding rates be modulated?

Catalysis of protein folding

Incorporating the influence of embedding contexts – epigenetic or chaperone effects, or the impact of (broadly) toxic exposures – can be done here by invoking the joint asymptotic equipartition theorem (Cover and Thomas, 2006). For example, given an embedding contextual information source, say Z, that affects protein development, then the developmental source uncertainty H_{G_i} is replaced by a joint uncertainty $H(X_{G_i}, Z)$. The objects of interest then become the jointly typical dual sequences $y^n = (x^n, z^n)$, where x is associated with protein folding development and z with the embedding context. Restricting consideration of x and z to those sequences that are in fact jointly typical allows use of the information transmitted from Z to X as the splitting criterion.

One important inference is that, from the information theory 'chain rule' (Cover and Thomas, 2006),

$$H(X, Z) \leq H(X) + H(Z),$$

so that the effect of the interactive embedding context, in this model, is to lower the *relative* free energy of a particular physically instantiated protein channel, analogous to the metabolic constraints described in Section 2.3.

Thus, the effect of epigenetic/catalytic regulation or toxic exposure is to channel protein folding into pathways that might otherwise be inhibited or slowed by an energy barrier. Hence, the epigenetic/catalytic/toxic information source Z acts as a *tunable catalyst*, a kind of second order enzyme, to enable and direct developmental pathways.

This is indeed a relative energy argument, since, metabolically, two systems must now be supported, i.e., that of the 'reaction' itself and that of its catalytic regulator. 'Programming' and stabilizing inevitably intertwined, as it were, a matter that will become central to questions of 'side effects' in the context of medical multifactorial 'magic strategy' interventions.

Protein folding, in the developmental picture, can be visualized as a series of branching pathways. Each branch point is a developmental decision, or switch point, governed by some regulatory apparatus (if only the slope of the folding funnel) that may include the effects of toxins or epigenetic mechanisms.

A more general picture emerges by allowing a distribution of possible 'final' states $\mathbf{S}_f$. The groupoid arguments merely expand to permit traverse of both initial states and possible final sets, recognizing that there can now be a possible overlap in the latter, and the catalytic effects are realized through the joint uncertainties $H(X_{G_i}, Z)$, so that the guiding information source Z serves to direct as well the possible final states of X_{G_i}.

Extending the model

The most natural extension of the developmental model of protein folding would be in terms of the directed homotopy classification of ontological trajectories, in the sense of Wallace and Wallace (2008, 2009). That is, developmental trajectories themselves can be classified into equivalence classes, for example, those that lead to a normal final state $\mathbf{S}_f$, and those that lead to pathological aggregations or misfoldings, say some set $\{\mathbf{S}_{path}^i\}, i = 1, 2, \ldots$. This produces a dynamic directed homotopy groupoid topology whose understanding might be useful across a broad spectrum of diseases.

Figure 6.1 illustrates the concept. The initial developmental state $\mathbf{S}_0$ can, in this picture, 'fall' down two different sets of developmental pathways, separated by a critical period 'shadow' preventing crossover between them. Paths within one set can be topologically transformed into each other without crossing the filled triangle, and constitute directed homotopy equivalence classes. The lower apex of the triangle can, however, start at many possible critical period points along any path connecting $\mathbf{S}_0$ and $\mathbf{S}_f$, following the arguments of Section 12 of Wallace and Wallace (2009).

Onset of a path that converges on the conformation $\mathbf{S}_{path}$ is, according to the model, driven by a genetic, epigenetic, or environmental catalysis event, in the sense of Fig. 2.1. The topological equivalence classes define a groupoid on the developmental system.

6.6 A Comprehensive Treatment

It is now possible to take the developmental perspective as the foundation for generating an empirically-based statistical model – effectively a cognitive paradigm for protein folding – that explicitly incorporates the embedding contexts of epigenetic and environmental signals. The argument is familiar.

A pattern of incoming input $\mathbf{S}_i$ describing the folding status of the protein – starting with the initial codon stream $\mathbf{S}_0$ of Section 6.5 – is mixed in a systematic algorithmic manner with a pattern of otherwise unspecified 'ongoing activity', including cellular, epigenetic and environmental signals,

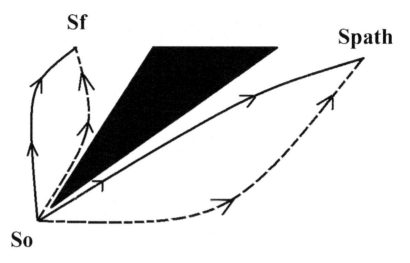

Fig. 6.1   Given an initial state $\mathbf{S}_0$ and a critical period casting a path-dependent developmental shadow, there are two different directed homotopy equivalence classes of deformable paths leading, respectively, to the normal folded protein state $\mathbf{S}_f$ and the pathological state $\mathbf{S}_{path}$. These sets of paths form equivalence classes defining a topological groupoid.

$\mathbf{W}_i$, to create a path of combined signals $x = (a_0, a_1, ..., a_n, ...)$.   Each a_k thus represents some functional composition of internal and external factors, and is expressed in terms of the intermediate states as

$$\mathbf{S}_{i+1} = f([\mathbf{S}_i, \mathbf{W}_i]) = f(a_i) \qquad (6.8)$$

for some unspecified function f. The a_i are seen to be very complicated composite objects in this treatment that we may choose to coarse-grain so as to obtain an appropriate 'alphabet'.

In a simple spinglass-like model, $\mathbf{S}$ would be a vector, $\mathbf{W}$ a matrix, and f would be a function of their product at 'time' i.

Following closely the argument of Section 1.3, the path x is fed into a highly nonlinear decision function, h, a 'sudden threshold machine' pattern recognition structure, in a sense, that generates an output $h(x)$ that is an element of one of two disjoint sets B_0 and B_1 of possible system responses. Let us define the sets B_k as

$$B_0 = \{b_0, ..., b_k\},$$

$$B_1 = \{b_{k+1}, ..., b_m\}.$$

Assume, as in Section 1.3, a graded response, supposing that if $h(x) \in B_0$, the pattern is not recognized, and if $h(x) \in B_1$, the pattern has been recognized, and some action $b_j, k + 1 \leq j \leq m$ takes place. Typically, the set B_1 would represent the final state of the folded protein, either normal or in some pathological conformation, that is sent on in the biological process or else subjected to some attempted corrective action. Corrections may, for example, range from activation of 'heat shock' protein repair to more drastic clean-up attack.

The principal objects of formal interest are paths x triggering pattern recognition-and-response. That is, given a fixed initial state $a_0 = [\mathbf{S}_0, \mathbf{W}_0]$, examine all possible subsequent paths x beginning with a_0 and leading to the event $h(x) \in B_1$. Thus, $h(a_0, ..., a_j) \in B_0$ for all $0 < j < m$, but $h(a_0, ..., a_m) \in B_1$. B_1 is thus the set of final possible states, $\{\mathbf{S}_f\} \cup \{\mathbf{S}_{path}\}$ from Fig. 6.1 that includes both the final 'physics' state $\mathbf{S}_f$ and the set of possible pathological conformations.

Again, for each positive integer n, let $N(n)$ be the number of high probability grammatical and syntactical paths of length n which begin with some particular a_0 and lead to the condition $h(x) \in B_1$. Call such paths 'meaningful', assuming – again – that $N(n)$ will be considerably less than the number of all possible paths of length n leading from a_0 to the condition $h(x) \in B_1$.

To reiterate, while the combining algorithm, the form of the nonlinear decision function h, and the details of grammar and syntax, can all be unspecified in this model, the critical assumption that permits inference of the necessary conditions constrained by the asymptotic limit theorems of information theory is that the finite limit $H = \lim_{n \to \infty} \log[N(n)]/n$ both exists and is independent of the path x.

In the terminology of Section 1.3, again call such a pattern recognition-and-response cognitive process *ergodic*. Not all cognitive processes are likely to be ergodic in this sense, implying that H, if it indeed exists at all, is path dependent, although extension to nearly ergodic processes appears possible (Wallace and Fullilove, 2008).

Invoking the spirit of the Shannon–McMillan theorem, as choice involves an inherent reduction in uncertainty, it is then possible to define an adiabatically, piecewise stationary, ergodic (APSE) information source, in the sense of Section 1.3, $\mathbf{X}$ associated with stochastic variates X_j having joint and conditional probabilities $P(a_0, ..., a_n)$ and $P(a_n | a_0, ..., a_{n-1})$ such that appropriate conditional and joint Shannon uncertainties satisfy the classic relations of Eq. (1.2).

This is, again, the dual information source to the underlying cognitive process.

Structure is now subsumed within the sequential grammar and syntax of the dual information source rather than within the set of developmental paths of Fig. 6.1 and the added catalysis arguments of Section 6.5.

This transformation in perspective carries heavy computational burdens, as well as providing deeper mathematical insight, as cellular machineries, and phenomena of epigenetic or environmental catalysis, are now included within a single model.

The energy and development pictures of Sections 6.4 and 6.5 were 'dual' as simply different aspects of the convexity of the rate distortion function with average distortion. This model seems qualitatively different, invoking a 'black box' information theory statistical model involving grammar and syntax driven by an asymptotic limit theorem, the Shannon–McMillan theorem.

The set of nonequilibrium empirical generalized Onsager models derived from it, as in Chapter 3, is based on the information source uncertainty H as a free energy-analog, thus having a significantly different meaning from those above, and are more similar to regression models fitted according to the central limit theorem. In a manner similar to the treatment in Wallace (2005), the system becomes subject to 'biological' renormalizations at critical, highly punctuated, transitions.

The most evident assumption at this point is that there may be more than a single cognitive protein folding process in operation, e.g., that the action of chaperones and other corrective mechanisms involve separate cognitive processes $\{H_1, ..., H_m\}$ that interact via crosstalk. Taking the direction of Chapter 3, there follows a complicated version of an internal system of empirical Onsager equations, assuming that the different cognitive processes represented by these dual information sources *become each other's primary environments*, a broadly, if locally, coevolutionary phenomenon, in the sense of Champagnat *et al.* (2006). Then

$$H_k = H_k(K_1, ..., K_s, ..., H_j, ...,), \qquad (6.9)$$

where the K_s represent other relevant parameters and $k \neq j$. In a generalization of the statistical model, we would expect the dynamics of such a system to be driven by an empirical recursive network of stochastic differential equations. Letting the K_s and H_j all be represented as parameters Q_j, with the caveat that H_k not depend on itself, define an entropy-analog based on the homology of information source uncertainty with free energy as the Legendre transform

$$S_k = H_k - \sum_i Q_i \partial H_k / \partial Q_i \,, \qquad (6.10)$$

whose gradients in the Q_j define local (broadly) chemical forces. In close analogy with other nonequilibrium phenomena, as described in Chapter 3, it becomes possible to invoke a complicated recursive system of phenomenological Onsager relation stochastic differential equations:

$$dQ_t^j = \sum_i [L_{j,i}(t, ..., Q_k, ...)dt + \sigma_{j,i}(t, ..., Q_k, ...)dB_t^i] \,, \qquad (6.11)$$

where, again, for notational simplicity, both parameters and information sources are expressed in terms of the same symbols Q^k. The dB_t^i represent different kinds of 'noise' having particular forms of quadratic variation that may represent a projection of environmental factors.

The Mathematical Appendix provides an introduction to stochastic differential equations via the Martingale theorem.

As described in Chapter 3, there can be multiple quasi-stable points within a given system's $\{..., H_k..., ..., K_j, ...\}$ representing a class of generalized resilience modes (Holling, 1973; Gunderson, 2000) accessible via punctuation as various possible outcomes of the protein folding process: normal, repaired, eliminated, and pathological. These topological states can, in theory, be found by setting the analytic Eq. (6.11) to zero, as the noise terms preclude unstable equilibria.

The essential point is that, under resilience theory, 'perturbations' of various sorts can be expected to shift the system between different quasi-stable folding modes, and, once shifted, correction may be exceedingly difficult or impossible, as these are, broadly, developmental processes having significant path dependence.

From a therapeutic perspective, medical intervention can be represented in terms of a 'large deviation' having the form of Eq. (3.5) that could, in theory, return pathological protein developmental paths to a more normal state. This will, in fact, be the central theme of Chapter 10.

6.7 Aging and Protein Folding

The developmental perspective above, although focused on the relatively short time frames of protein metabolism – in the range from microseconds to minutes – is suggestive. The principal 'risk factor' for a large array of protein folding disorders is biological age – for humans, in the range of decades – and a simplified version of the previous section may provide a life-course perspective, that is, a developmental model over a far longer timescale.

The rate distortion function, $R(D)$, is itself a free energy measure, as it represents the minimum channel capacity needed to assure average distortion equal to or less than D. Let us now consider the principal branch in Fig. 6.1, the set of paths from $\mathbf{S}_0$ to $\mathbf{S}_f$, representing normal protein folding, taken as a communication channel having a given rate distortion function. The arguments of Section 3.2 suggest that there will be an empirical Onsager equation in the gradient of the rate distortion disorder, an entropy-analog Legendre transform

$$S_R \equiv R(D) - DdR(D)/dD,\qquad(6.12)$$

such that, over a life-history timeline,

$$dD/dt = f(dS_R/dD)\qquad(6.13)$$

for some appropriate function f.

Recall the development of Section 3.2: for a Gaussian channel, having $R(D) = (1/2)\log[\sigma^2/D]$,

$$S_R(D) = (1/2)\log[\sigma^2/D] + 1/2,$$

and the simplest possible Onsager equation becomes

$$dD/dt = -\mu dS_R dD = \frac{\mu}{2D},\qquad(6.14)$$

with the explicit solution

$$D = \sqrt{\mu t}.\qquad(6.15)$$

For an appropriate timescale – necessarily many orders of magnitude longer than the time of folding itself – the average distortion, representing the degree of misfolding, simply grows as a diffusion process in time. This is the simplest possible aging model, in which μ represents the rate of accumulating epigenetic and broadly environmental effects including toxic exposures, nutrition, the richness of social interaction, and so on, over a lifetime.

A somewhat less simplistic model takes the Onsager relation as constrained by the availability of metabolic free energy, M, that powers active chaperone processes,

$$dD/dt = -\mu dS_R/dD - \kappa M = \frac{\mu}{2D} - \kappa M,\qquad(6.16)$$

where κ represents the efficiency of use of metabolic energy. Again, this equation has the equilibrium solution (i.e., when $dD/dt = 0$)

$$D_{equlib} = \frac{\mu}{2\kappa M} .$$ (6.17)

Here, aging is represented by a decay in the efficiency of those chaperone processes, i.e., a slow decline in κ, that may involve idiosyncratic dynamics, ranging from punctuated phase transitions to autocatalytic runaway effects, since D, in Eq. (6.2), acts as a temperature analog for a system able to undergo symmetry breaking.

6.8   Summary

The fidelity of the translation between genome and final protein conformation, measured by an average distortion measure, or its dual, the minimum channel capacity needed to limit average distortion to a given level, serve as evolutionarily sculpted temperature analogs, in the sense of Onuchic and Wolynes (2004), to determine the possible phase transitions defining different degrees of protein symmetry. The protein folding funnel follows a spontaneous symmetry breaking mechanism with average distortion as the temperature analog, or, in the developmental picture, greater channel capacity that leads more directly to the final state $\mathbf{S}_f$.

The various outcomes to the full protein folding process – normal, corrected, eliminated, pathological – emerge, in the expanded 'Onsager' statistical model based on a cognitive paradigm, as distinct 'resilience' modes of a complicated internal cellular ecosystem, subject to punctuated transitions driven, in some cases, by signals from embedding epigenetic and ecological structures. Increase in the rate of folding disorders with age emerges through a long-time generalization of the Onsager model.

In a sense this work extends Tlusty's (2007) elegant topological exploration of the evolution of the genetic code, suggesting that rate distortion considerations are central to a broad spectrum of molecular biological phenomena, although different measures may come to the fore under different perspectives.

The cognitive paradigm introduced here opens a unified biological vision of protein folding and its disorders that may relate the etiology of a large set of misfolding and aggregation diseases more clearly to both cellular and epigenetic processes and environmental stressors. This would be, in the current reductionist sandstorm, no small thing. A cognitive paradigm subsumes epigenetic and environmental catalysis of protein conformation 'development' within a single grammar and syntax, and allows both normal folding and its pathologies to both be viewed as 'natural' outcomes, a perspective more consistent with rates of folding and aggregation disorders observed within an aging population.

Most basically, however, such a cognitive paradigm – viewing protein folding regulation as part of the larger human cognome – serves as the foundation for a new class of statistical tools based on the asymptotic limit theorems of information theory, rather than on the central limit theorem alone, that should be useful in the analysis of data related to protein misfolding and aggregation disorders.

Chapter 7

EXAMPLE: GLYCOME DETERMINANTS

7.1 Introduction

Glycomics is the study of the glycans and glycoconjugates – loosely, carbo-hydrates – produced by a cell or organism under specific conditions (e.g., Hart and Copeland, 2010). The glycome – the general body of such sub-stances – is not well characterized. Mian and Rose (2011), for example, write that:

> Superficially, the paucity of information- and coding-theoretic studies of carbohydrates can be explained by glycomics being a less mature field than genomics or proteonics... A deeper explanation is the more complex and dynamic nature of the glycome – the entire complement of carbohydrates... of an organism or a cell... Commu-nication theoretic studies of the glycome and the [glycan code], the complex information conveyed by glycans and glycoconjugates, would increase understanding of the major events in macroevolution and ex-tant molecular biology. For example, the biological communication mediated by glycans underlies diverse molecular, cellular, and tissue functions and plays critical roles in development, health and disease.

Tlusty (2007, 2008) examines the production of amino acids from codons via an information-theoretic index theorem formulation based on applica-tion of topological methods to a network error analysis, an approach that can be used to illuminate something of the difficulties currently facing gly-comics.

Wallace (2010a, 2011a) has, in fact, applied Tlusty's methods to struc-tured protein folding, and it is possible, in some measure, to extend that work to the glycome. The fundamental problem, however, is that both gene coding for amino acids, and many processes of protein folding, can be described as deterministic-but-for-errors. As Anfinsen (1973) has shown, an amino acid 'string' for a structured protein carries within it the information needed for correct folding, at least at near-zero aqueous concentrations of metabolites. The Hecht group (e.g., Hecht *et al.*, 2004; Kim and Hecht, 2006) has shown that the famous protein α-helices and β-sheets are simply 'coded' by strings of alternating hydrophobic and hydrophilic amino acids having the digital signal forms 101100100110... and 101010101... respectively, where 1 indicates polar and 0 non-polar amino acid. The α-helix thus has a 3.6 residue/turn pattern, and the β-sheets alternate. Any polar/nonpolar amino acids will suffice, although folding rates will vary greatly, and this degeneracy permits application of Tlusty's error analysis. Glycans are different, as Hart and Copeland (2010) explain:

Unlike nucleic acids and proteins, glycan structures are not hardwired into the genome, depending upon a template for their synthesis. Rather, the glycan structures that end up on a polypeptide or lipid result from the concerted actions of highly specific glycosyltransferases...which are in turn dependent upon [a multiplicity of other processes]... Therefore, the glycoforms of a glycoprotein depend on many factors directly tied to both gene expression and cellular metabolism.

Chapters 4 and 5 explored, in some measure, a cognitive paradigm for gene expression that involves channeling by environmental and developmental signals to turn genes on or off. More detail can be found in Wallace and Wallace (2008, 2009, 2010). Chapter 6 examined protein folding regulation. This chapter extends that work to the glycome, again using the fact that a broad class of cognitive processes can be represented by dual information sources, permitting an ultimate generalization of Tlusty's methods via the asymptotic limit theorems of information theory.

After a brief recapitulation of Tlusty's work, it becomes possible to concisely state the 'central problem' of glycomics from that perspective, and to describe a strategy of theoretical attack loosely based on the rate distortion manifold approach of Glazebrook and Wallace (2009a, b). What emerges is a process of cellular chemical cognition whose description via topological operator methods leads to an elaborate 'spectral decomposition' that – finally – generalizes Tlusty's approach, albeit in second order.

This modeling exercise suggests that reductionist descriptions of glycan process and dysfunction may not be appropriate, in the context of diverse chains of sophisticated chemical cognition that appear to be more difficult to understand than even high order neural cognition (e.g., Wallace, 2005, 2007).

7.2 Stochastic Topology

Tlusty (2007) describes the genetic code in terms of an error-network of equivalent and nearly-equivalent codons:

> The maximum [of a particular information-theory-based Morse function] determines a single contiguous domain where a certain amino acid is encoded... Thus every mode [of the network] corresponds to an amino acid and the number of modes is the number of amino acids. This compact organization is advantageous because misreading of one codon as another codon within the same domain has no deleterious impact. For example, if the code has two amino acids, it is evident that the error-load of an arrangement where there are two large contiguous regions, each coding for a different amino acid, is much smaller than a 'checkerboard' arrangement of the amino acids.

This, Tlusty points out (2010), is analogous, but not identical, to the well-known topological coloring problem: "in the coding problem one desires maximal similarity in the colors of neighboring 'countries', while in the coloring problem one must color neighboring countries by different colors". After some development (Tlusty, 2008), the number of possible amino acids in this error manifold scheme is determined by Heawood's formula (Ringel and Young, 1968), an *index theorem*, in the sense of Hazewinkel (2002), that relates topological to analytic properties:

$$chr(\gamma) = int(\frac{1}{2}(7 + \sqrt{1 + 48\gamma})), \qquad (7.1)$$

where $chr(\gamma)$ is the number of color domains of a surface with genus γ – roughly the number of holes in the surface – and $int(x)$ is the integer value of x.

From Morse theory (e.g., Matsumoto, 2002), there is another important index theorem relating topology to the analytical structure of a manifold:

$$\gamma = 1 - \frac{1}{2}\chi, \qquad (7.2)$$

where χ is the Euler characteristic of the underlying topological manifold. For a manifold having a Morse function f, χ can be expressed as the alternating sum of the function's Morse numbers: the Morse numbers $\mu_i (i = 0, 1, ..., m)$ of f on the manifold are the number of critical points $(df(x_c) = 0)$ of index i, the number of negative eigenvalues of the matrix $H_{i,j} = \partial f^2 / \partial x_i \partial x_j$. Then $\chi = \sum_{i=0}^{m} (-1)^i \mu_i$. This holds true for any Morse function on the manifold M.

Part of Tlusty's Table 1, showing the topological limit to the number of amino acids for different codes, is given below:

Code	# Codons	Max. # AA's
4-base singlets	4	4
3-base doublets	9	7
4-base doublets	16	11
16 codons	32	16
48 codons	48	20
4-base triplets	64	25

This is the fundamental topological decomposition, to which Morse theory 'free energy' functionals, like Tlusty's, are to be fit.

Wallace (2010a, 2011a) has applied Tlusty's method to the classification of protein symmetries, deriving the underlying topology of the 'protein folding error code' from the observed number of canonical protein conformations. Following the seminal work of Levitt and Chothia (1976), there are four major globular protein structures: all-α helices, all-β sheets, α/β, $\alpha + \beta$, with obvious definitions. Chou and Maggioria (1998), using heroic methods on a much larger data set, identify a total of from seven to ten such classes, the majority of which seem fairly rare. From the table below, that displays Eq. (7.1), the normal globular 'protein folding code error network', in Tlusty's sense, is essentially a large connected 'sphere' – giving the four dominant structures – having one minor, and possibly as many as three more 'subminor' attachment handles in the Morse theory sense (Matsumoto, 2002).

γ (# network holes)	chr(γ) (# symmetries)
0	4
1	7
2	8
3	9
4	10
5	11
6, 7	12
8, 9	13

7.3   The Glycomic Conundrum

As adapted from Gupta *et al.* (2010), Fig. 7.1 schematically illustrates the exponential progression in information content from the genome to the mammalian glycome. Genomic and protein structures are template driven. By contrast, glycome signaling structures are finger-like projections of a characteristic number of basic monosaccharides and side chains whose contingent expression is dependent on a complicated, shifting, cascade of processes.

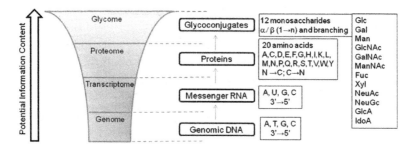

Fig. 7.1   Adapted from Fig. 1 of Gupta *et al.* (2010). There is an exponential increase in the amount of potential information content from the genome through the proteome up to the glycome. The basic monosaccharides – 12 for the mammalian glycome – form branches with side chains that may represent as many as 10,000 glycan determinant 'amino acids'.

It is of some importance to note that the production of the 12 mammalian monosaccharides fits into a basic scheme of an underlying Tlusty-style error code network having, according to the table above, six or seven topological holes. These numbers may vary considerably across eukaryotes, prokaryotes, and archaea, but are likely to fit Heawood's classification scheme. However, in all cases, as Richard Cummings (2009) reviews, the major classes of glycan determinants recognized by glycan-binding proteins are in the branches made up of these basic components, i.e., the tips of carbohydrates on cellular surfaces that are recognized by other chemical species. It is here that the essential business of signaling actually takes place.

These tips are made up of two to six linear monosaccharides together with their potential side chains containing other sugars and modifications like sulfonation, phosphorylation, and acetylation. Glycosaminoglycans comprise repeating disaccharide motifs, where a linear sequence of five to six monosaccharides may be required for recognition. Cummings estimates that human glycoproteins and glycolipids may contain a minimum of 3,000 glycan determinants, with an additional minimum of 4,000 theoretical polysaccharide sequences in glycosaminoglycans, say a total of 7,000–10,000 glycan determinants. Figure 7.2 applies Heawood's formula to the case of 10,000 'amino acids': the underlying 'glycome code error network' must be a grossly complicated topological object (GCTO), having between 4 and 8 million holes.

In essence, any idea of a biologically real 'glycan code' analogous to the genetic code fails spectacularly through this *reductio ad absurdum.*

The solution to this extraordinary ambiguity is precisely similar to that of the gene expression problem, where external signals guide the timing of turning some tens of thousands of genes on and off during development to produce a vast array of appropriate phenotypes: incoming information limits and channels development (Wallace and Wallace, 2008, 2009, 2010). That is, even the *in vitro* genetic code is defined *in vivo* by the influence of an elaborate gene expression regulatory apparatus. Here, we simply proceed to regulation in the absence of a well-defined 'code', although its ghost serves as a kind of zero-order starting point for more elaborate analyses.

7.4   Another Cognitive Paradigm

To reiterate, the glycoforms of a glycoprotein depend on many factors directly tied to both gene expression and cellular metabolism. This suggests the operation of a cellular-level process of chemical cognition, broadly analogous to the operation of the immune system as described by Atlan and Cohen (1998). Thus, incoming information 'farms' glycoforms, in the context of available metabolic energy intensity.

It is possible – albeit rather artificially – to envision an initial two-step approach, first exploring the effects of incoming signals that limit consideration to a subsection of the GCTO of the 'glycan error network'. Another step is needed to actually produce and regulate the appropriate glycan determinant from the chosen subset of code. The argument becomes, not uncharacteristically, progressively more complicated as constraints increase.

In reality, this is a single elaborate process of chemical cognition carried out via the endoplasmic reticulum, the Golgi apparatus, and associated structures.

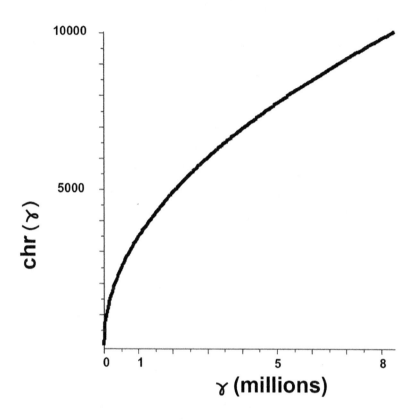

Fig. 7.2 Heawood's topological coloring formula: the number of glycan determinant modes analogous to amino acids is shown vs. number of 'holes' in the underlying error network manifold. The 10,000 modes representing Cummings' human glycan determinants require an underlying error network with 8.3 million holes. More complicated topological schemes for other taxa would be correspondingly larger.

The dual information source

Cognition – here, taken as the selection of a small part of the GCTO for actual implementation – involves choice that limits uncertainty, and thus a broad class of cognitive processes can be represented by 'dual' information sources. The underlying model, again, follows Atlan and Cohen (1998) and generalizes the results of Wallace (2000), as has been described at length in the previous chapters.

Again, cognitive pattern recognition-and-selected response, from this perspective, proceeds by systematically mixing an incoming external 'sensory' signal with an internal 'ongoing activity' – which includes, but is not limited to, some learned or inherited picture of the world – and, at some point, triggering an appropriate action based on a decision that the pattern of sensory activity requires a response. It is not necessary to specify how the pattern recognition system is trained, and hence possible to adopt a 'weak' model, applicable regardless of learning paradigm. Fulfilling Atlan and Cohen's criterion of meaning-from-response, it is possible to define a language's contextual meaning entirely in terms of system output, as in the earlier chapters.

The central function of the cognitive chemical selection process defined here is to restrict the play of the information-theoretic Morse function, in Tlusty's sense, whose modes define the amino acid analogs of the 10,000 glycan determinants – to choose what is to be produced.

The essential point is that the dual information source representing the cognitive selection of some small zone of the GCTO is itself acted on by gene expression and metabolic contexts. Cognitive gene expression, in the sense of Wallace and Wallace (2008, 2009), can be represented by impinging dual information sources. It is this interaction that 'corrects', in a sense, the fiction of a 'glycan error code network', taken as a conceptual starting point for this analysis.

Again, the tools for the action of such external context on the GCTO selector is network information theory (e.g., Cover and Thomas, 2006; El Gamal and Kim, 2010), in the context of the information theory chain rule. To reiterate, given three interacting information sources, Y_1, Y_2, Z, the splitting criterion for tripartite jointly typical sequences, taking Z as an external context, is (Cover and Thomas, 2006, p. 524)

$$I(Y_1; Y_2|Z) = H(Z) + H(Y_1|Z) + H(Y_2|Z) - H(Y_1, Y_2, Z) \leq$$
$$H(Z) + H(Y_1) + H(Y_2), \quad (7.3)$$

where $H(...|...)$ and $H(..., ..., ...)$ represent conditional and joint uncertainties, and the second line is an example of the 'information chain rule' (Ash, 1990; Khinchin, 1957; Cover and Thomas, 2006).

Since information is a form of free energy instantiated by physical processes that require massive intensities of metabolic free energy, at the expense of maintaining three information sources – Z, Y_1 and Y_2 – it is thus possible to canalize $I(Y_1; Y_2|Z)$ in such a manner as to make a desired patch of the GCTO the lowest relative energy state. Previous chapters use similar methods.

More complicated multivariate typical sequences receive much the same treatment (El Gamel and Kim, 2010). Given a basic set of information sources $(X_1, ..., X_k)$ that one partitions into two ordered sets $X(J)$ and $X(J')$, then the splitting criterion becomes $H(X(J)|X(J'))$. Generalization is straightforward.

Then, the joint splitting criterion – I, H above – however expressed as a composite of the underlying information sources and their interactions, satisfies a relation analogous to Eq. (1.3), where $N(n)$ is the number of high probability jointly typical paths of length n. The joint splitting criterion is given as a functional composition of the underlying information sources and their interactions as affected by the embedding contextual cognitive information sources indexed by J', and canalization follows from the information theory chain rule.

In reality, there will most likely be a large ensemble of possible reaction trajectories, and one must take a statistical approach. That is, letting $< ... >$ represent an averaging process,

$$[< I >] < \sum_j < H_j > . \tag{7.4}$$

Given an index of available metabolic free energy intensity M_j for each information source, the average becomes

$$< H_j >= \frac{\int H_j \exp[-H_j/\kappa M_j]dH_j}{\int \exp[-H_j/\kappa M_j]dH_j} \approx \kappa M_j , \tag{7.5}$$

where κ is an appropriate scaling constant, expected to be very small indeed as a consequence of entropic translation losses.

Then

$$M_I < \sum_j M_j , \tag{7.6}$$

and, again, this provides an explicit free energy mechanism for reaction canalization.

That is, entropic translation losses – $M_j \gg H_j$ – can actually be a tool for triggering complex biological logic gates, in much the sense that Tompa and Csermely (2004) propose that entropy transfer can be used by generalized chaperones to trigger proper structure in pathologically folded protein complexes.

7.5   Regulating Glycan Determinants

As described in the previous chapter, although a large class of protein fold-ing is, following Anfinsen's (1973) elegant studies *in vitro*, deterministic in aqueous context at vanishingly low concentrations of metabolites, *in vivo* it is well known amyloid and other pathological conformations compete ther-modynamically with the 'protein folding code': protein folding disorders such as Alzheimer's disease are ubiquitous.

Thus, the endoplasmic reticulum and related structures embody an elab-orate chemical cognitive regulatory process that chaperones, repairs, or eliminates misfolded strings of amino acids. It seems obvious that the pro-duction of glycan determinants, once the cognitive fovea limiting focus on the GCTO has determined what is to be produced, can be no less rigorously regulated. Analysis requires the introduction of rate distortion arguments.

Think of the machinery focusing on a subset of the GCTO as communi-cating with machinery that produces and places the glycan determinants. Suppose it possible to compare what is actually produced with what should have been produced, perhaps by a simple evolutionary survival mechanism, perhaps via some more sophisticated evolutionarily driven error-correcting systems generating another 'funnel' construct. This leads directly to rate distortion conditions, in the sense of the Mathematical Appendix.

Consider, now, developmental pathways in a 'phenotype space' that, in a series of steps, take a cognitively selected 'glycan codon-like' message – $\mathbf{S}_0$ at time 0 – to the final glycan determinant-in-context $\mathbf{S}_f$ in a sequence of intermediate configurations. What are the dynamics of the process? The simplest approach again makes use of the convex nature of $R(D)$ in an analog to Onsager's nonequilibrium thermodynamics.

Interpreting the rate distortion function as another form of free energy suggests again defining a rate distortion entropy S_R in some set of param-eters $\mathbf{Q} = \{Q_1, ..., Q_k\}$, where $Q_1 \equiv D$, as the Legendre transform

$$S_R \equiv R(\mathbf{Q}) - \sum_j Q_j dR(\mathbf{Q})/dQ_j . \qquad (7.7)$$

The Onsager formalism defines chemical forces in terms of gradients in entropy (e.g., de Groot and Mazur, 1984), so that we write, for example,

$$dQ_j/dt = \sum_k L_{j,k} dS_R(\mathbf{Q})/dQ_k . \qquad (7.8)$$

As discussed previously, a locally time-reversible system will have $L_{i,j} = L_{j,i}$. For information sources this is not appropriate: palindromes are rare.

Equation (7.8) generalizes to the usual set of stochastic differential equations

$$dQ_j = \sum_k [L_{j,k}(t, \mathbf{Q})dt + \sigma_{j,k}(t, \mathbf{Q})dB_t^k]\,, \qquad (7.9)$$

where the 'noise' terms B^k are characterized by their quadratic variation.

Setting this equation to zero again generates an index theorem relating topology to the solution of an analytic equation.

7.6 Glycan Spectra

Figure 7.3, adapted from Cohen and Varki (2010), shows the hierarchy of increasing complexity in glycan structure, from, in this case, sialic acid leaves-and-flowers to sialylated microdomains on a membrane surface. It is possible to define a chemical operator whose discrete spectrum represents these microdomains. This 'topological quantization' represents an extension of a complicated stack of phenomena that must include elaborate regulatory processes of chemical cognition.

The argument is both familiar and direct. From the discussion above, it is clear there is a necessary dependence on maximum allowable average distortion in a topological patch-mapping process $\mathbf{T}[\{\mathbf{S}_0\}] \rightarrow \{\mathbf{S}_f\}$. Setting Eq. (7.9) to zero again produces an index theorem in the sense of Section 3.1 that relates the solutions of an analytic equation to the underlying set of topological structures represented by the topological mapping $\mathbf{T}[\{\mathbf{S}_0\}] \rightarrow \{\mathbf{S}_f\}$.

To see this, take the simplest first-order approximation as a polynomial dependence written as

$$G^n[\mu/D_{max}](\lambda) = 0\,, \qquad (7.10)$$

where n is the polynomial order, μ/D_{max} (from Eq. 6.17) is an index of metabolic free energy demand that depends inversely on the maximum allowed average distortion, and λ a measure of the topological complexity of the mapping. This produces $m \leq n$ possible microdomains that correspond to quasi-equilibria representing topological eigenmodes of the mapping operator. This is a familiar argument, but reached via a classical information theory approach replete with complicated regulatory processes of chemical cognition.

Many matters in glycomic theory now can, in this first order approximation, be reexpressed as questions regarding the eigenvalues and eigenmodes

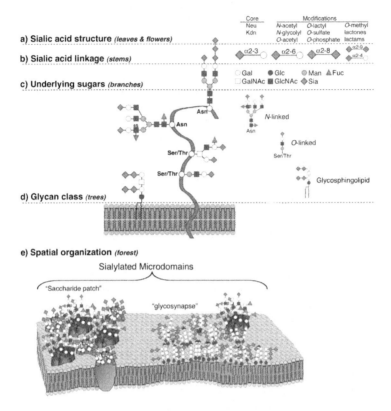

Fig. 7.3   Adapted from Cohen and Varki (2010). Hierarchical levels of sialome complexity, from core and core modifications at level (a) to spatially organized microdomains of clustered saccharide patches on membrane surfaces at level (e). These latter represent the mapping of initial to final state sets $\{S_0\} \to \{S_f\}$ via an operator having a spectrum representing different topological conformations. The structural hierarchy $(a) \to (e)$ suggests, in turn, a nested hierarchy of operators.

of an 'information operator' $\mathbf{T}$, and this seems, on the surface at least, a fairly familiar landscape.

Again, setting Eq. (7.9) to zero, and the simplified version of Eq. (7.10), are essentially index theorems analogous to Eqs. (7.1) and (7.2), and represent a further extension of Tlusty's method up the biological hierarchy, albeit in the context of complicated regulatory processes of chemical cognition. In that regard, as Hazewinkel (2002) comments, the 'index' need not be an integer, but may be a complex number or a function. Figure 7.3 suggests a nested hierarchy of operators $\mathbf{T}_a, ..., \mathbf{T}_e$, and such regularities should be observable.

The obvious conjecture is that, for different levels of the hierarchy of Fig. 7.3, n in Eq. (7.10) will be given by 'magic numbers' similar to (but perhaps quite different from) those of Heawood's formula, Eq. (7.1). An obvious extension is that, in setting Eq. (7.9) to zero so as to identify quasi-equilibria, the resulting functions can be approximated as 'stochastic polynomials' of finite order in the variables $\mathbf{Q}$. This is taken as the set of characteristic polynomials of an appropriate set of operators. More generally, however, as above, setting Eq. (7.9) equal to zero *directly* provides an index theorem in the sense of Atiyah and Singer (1963) that relates analytic results – the solutions to the equation – to an underlying set of topological structures, the 'eigenmodes of $\mathbf{T}$'.

Although information is a form of free energy, the operators $\mathbf{T}_k$ are finite dimensional, having well-defined, indeed, classical, topological eigenspaces. One suspects that other characteristics of the system can be used to define the relative probabilities of the different eigenmodes. For the protein folding case the four major classifications, i.e., $\alpha, \beta, \alpha + \beta$ and α/β, seem to have higher probabilities than the remaining sets of possible topological conformations. The question remains open.

What is clear is that different organisms, or tissues within organisms, will have markedly different 'glycan spectra', and that these spectra will have complicated dynamic properties dependent on interactions with embedding environments and interacting organisms. It appears that such glycan spectra are, for biology-as-we-know it, as characteristic and diverse as atomic, subatomic, and molecular spectra are in the physical sciences.

7.7   Summary

Where *in vivo* protein folding and its (manifold) disorders can be at least addressed via a one-stage regulatory model, courtesy of Anfinsen's (1973) deterministic *in vitro* observations, the production and placement of glycan determinants requires the synergistic cooperation of a chain of sophisticated phenomena of chemical cognition that must first identify a desired set of glycan determinants, and then both construct and shepherd the chosen species to their final physiologically active positions.

Intermediate topological regularities, analogous to the approximately fourfold globular protein classification, may well be found along this hierarchy of process, but the overall phenomenon seems to require fairly advanced mathematical tools for even an elementary sketch: index theorems are no small matter. Given the intellectual fog-of-war that surrounds protein folding and its disorders, the formal description of glycan process and dysfunction is going to be a very rough ride.

What seems to emerge, however, is that the regulation of 'low level' biochemical phenomena, ranging from gene expression and protein folding through the production of flexible glycan surface signaling fronds, increasingly appears to involve systems of chemical cognition that may fully rival the complexity of high order neural process.

The selection and regulation of the glycan determinants coating the cell surface – the system that, in fact, conveys most of the biological information available at the cellular level – is thus a principal module of the cognome.

Chapter 8

EXAMPLE: GLYCAN/LECTIN LOGIC GATES

8.1 Introduction

Figure 7.1, adapted from Gupta *et al.* (2010), illustrates the exponential increase in the amount of potential information content from the genome through the proteome up to the glycome. The 12 basic mammalian monosaccharides form branches with side chains that may represent 7,000 to 10,000 possible 'glycome determinants' (Cummings, 2009), forming larger structures that interact with lectin proteins to actually transmit biological information.

In vitro, punctuated transitions in glycan/lectin interaction topology cause large-scale phase change in reactions driven by experimental gradients in reactant concentration (Dam and Brewer, 2010). It is possible to adapt a phenomenological 'renormalization' strategy from statistical physics to such phase transitions. The essence of the argument is that information is a form of free energy, so that something resembling Wilson's (1971) renormalization methods can be abducted to complicated biological phase changes associated with biological information transmission. In an exactly parallel argument, perspectives abducted from nonrigid molecule theory suggest the possibility of elaborate symmetry breaking mechanisms, driven by indicies of overall topological structure. The two approaches appear as different aspects of the same elephant, as it were.

The transmission of information, however, inevitably involves a source that actually generates that information, something that 'speaks' a 'language', and such processes are constrained by the necessary conditions of the asymptotic limit theorems of information theory: the Shannon coding theorem, the Shannon–McMillan source coding theorem, and the rate distortion theorem, and variants like the information theory chain rule (Ash 1990; Cover and Thomas 2006; Khinchin 1957).

8.2   The Critical Exponent

For this work, the essential matter is the homology between information source uncertainty – the richness of the language being spoken – and the free energy density of a physical system. This allows adaptation of Wilson's (1971) renormalization symmetry methods for phase transitions.

Given an information source that produces as sequence of signals having structure – loosely, grammar and syntax – the Shannon–McMillan theorem says that such utterances can be broken into two disjoint parts, a very large set of gibberish that has vanishingly low probability, and a very small set in accordance with the rules of grammar and syntax characterizing the information source for which the following condition holds: in the now-familiar manner, let $N(n)$ be the number of grammatical and syntactical statements of length n produced by an information source X. Then the limit $H[X] = \lim_{n \to \infty} \log[N(n)]/n$ exists and is independent of the statement itself. That is, H is a universal constant for the information source. If the limit converges for some finite n_0, than that number is called the order of the information source.

A second limiting relation is that the statements produced by any information source must be transmitted along a channel having a channel capacity $C \geq 0$ such that $H[X] \leq C$.

Details can be found in any number of texts (Ash, 1990; Cover and Thomas, 2006; Khinchin, 1957).

Recall that the free energy density of a physical system having volume V and partition function $Z(\beta, V)$ derived from the system's Hamiltonian – the energy function – at normalized temperature β is (e.g., Landau and Lifshitz 2007)

$$F[\beta] = \lim_{V \to \infty} -\beta \frac{\log[Z(\beta, V)]}{V} \equiv$$

$$\lim_{V \to \infty} \frac{\log[\hat{Z}(\beta, V)]}{V},$$

with $\hat{Z} = Z^{-\beta}$.

The latter relation is formally similar to the expression above for H in terms of $\log[N(n)]/n$, a circumstance having deep implications. To reiterate, Feynman (2000) describes how information and free energy have an inherent duality, and defines information as the free energy needed to erase a message. Information is a form of free energy and the construction and transmission of information within living things consumes metabolic free energy, with inevitable – and massive – losses via the second law of thermodynamics.

It is possible to apply Wilson's (1971) famous renormalization strategy to characterize the behavior of channel capacity C near critical values of driving parameters. The basic argument is well known (e.g., Binney *et al.*, 1992): above and below the critical value of some driving parameter, say Tc, the system of interest has two distinct phases, characterized by an order parameter that vanishes above Tc. Take an empirical index of channel capacity as the order parameter. Let

$$\tau \equiv \frac{T - Tc}{Tc}.$$

The first term of a series expansion of C in τ, becomes

$$C(\tau) = A\tau^\alpha(1 + b\tau^{\alpha_1}...),$$

so that, in first order,

$$C(\tau) \propto \tau^\alpha.$$

A simple calculation gives

$$\alpha = \lim_{\tau \to 0} \frac{\log |C(\tau)|}{\log |\tau|}. \tag{8.1}$$

The hard trick is to calculate α from first principles. For (relatively) simple physical phenomena, such exponents are universal across many systems, a function of simple underlying renormalization symmetry relations (Wilson, 1971; Binney *et al.*, 1992). A detailed calculation in the Mathematical Appendix, however, shows that for biological structures, a vast array of 'biological' renormalizations are possible, and universality classes – collections of phenomena having the same α – may be limited to sets of very similar reacting species.

H and C, as free energy measures, can also be viewed as Morse functions, in the sense of Pettini (2007), and thus subject to the topological hypothesis: singularities in these measures – critical points – are to be associated with a fundamental change in underlying topology of the manifold on which these measures are defined. This is a generalization of Landau's observation (Landau and Lifshitz, 2007) that second-order phase transitions in simple physical systems, those without latent energy, are usually characterized by changes in underlying symmetry, with the higher energy states being more symmetric. It is possible to impose this perspective on glycan/lectin interaction.

8.3 Two Examples

Area concentration

The carbohydrate α-GalNAc interacts with the lectin biotinylated soybean agglutinin (SBA) in solution to form a sequence of increasingly complicated interlinked conformations at appropriate concentrations of reacting species. Dam *et al.* (2007) describe this 'bind-and-slide' process in terms of a change in topology, according to Fig. 8.1.

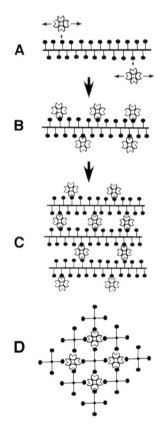

Fig. 8.1   Adapted from Dam *et al.* (2007). (A) At first, lectin diffuses along (and off) the glycan kelp frond, until, (B), a sufficient number of sites are occupied. Then (C), the lectin-coated glycan fronds begin to cross bind and the reaction is saturated. (D) shows an end-on view of the complex in (C).

Initially, the lectin diffuses along (and off) the glycan kelp frond, until a number of sites are occupied. Then the lectin-coated glycan fronds begin to cross bind, until the reaction saturates. Figure 8.1D shows an end-on view of the complex shown longitudinally in Fig. 8.1C.

Dam and Brewer (2008) generalize this as follows:

> The bind and slide model for lectins binding to multivalent glycosides, globular, and linear glycoproteins is distinct from the classical 'lock and key' model for ligand-receptor interactions. The bind and slide (internal diffusion) model allows a small fraction of bound lectin molecules to dynamically move from carbohydrate to carbohydrate epitope in globular and linear glycoproteins. This, in turn, can facilitate lectin-mediated cross-linking of such glycoproteins on the surface of cells... Such cross-linked receptors, in turn, trigger signal transduction mechanisms... Indeed, a large number of transmembrane receptors are found clustered... Thus the affinity and hence specificity of ligand-receptor interactions may be regulated by epitope and receptor clustering in many biological systems.

Under typical physiological circumstances, glycans form a literal kelp bed bound to cellular surfaces, and the essential (topological) 'intensity parameter' – the temperature analog – becomes area density of the fronds. The excellent review article of Dam and Brewer (2010) describes the work of Oyelaran *et al.* (2009), who conducted a series of heroic density-dependent fluorescence experiments, and it becomes possible to take the observed intensity of that fluorescence as an index of channel capacity, since no information transmission → no reaction → no fluorescence.

Using microarray methods, Oyelaran *et al.* embedded α-GalNAc onto bovine serum albumin (BSA), with different numbers of carbohydrate molecules (CM) per BSA site, typically ranging from 4 to 40. At density of 4, the CM were separated by about 85 Angstroms, and at 20, by about 40 Angstroms.

Typically, fluorescence intensity, K, under such conditions, follows a relation

$$K = \frac{Km}{Kd/L + 1}, \tag{8.2}$$

where Km is the maximum intensity, Kd the apparent dissociation constant for interaction between protein and immobilized glycoconjugate, and L the concentration of lectin. See Fig. 8.2.

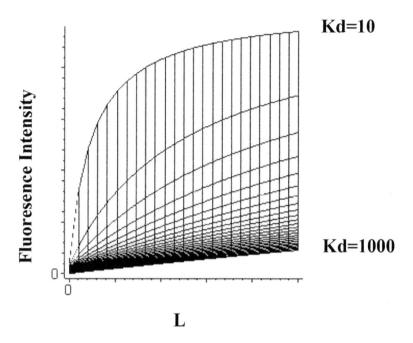

Fig. 8.2   Fluorescence intensity vs. lectin concentration for different values of Kd. Large Kd implies little fluorescence, and hence, by our arguments, small channel capacity, C.

The essential matter is the way in which Kd varies with glycan area density. For α-GalNAc embedded on BSA, again reacting with biotinylated soybean agglutinin, SBA, Kd followed the relation of Fig. 8.3.

Kd in Eq. (8.2) almost disappears with increasing number of glycan molecules per BSA site: the value falls from near 4,200 at $n=4$ to 194 at $n=9$, so that Kd is, from a physics perspective, an 'order parameter' that undergoes a change representing a topological transformation, here a cross-linking phase transition.

Volume concentration

As described by by Dam and Brewer (2010), classic work by Orr *et al.* (1979) examined aggregation of lecithin liposomes having a synthetic mannose glycolipid by concanavalin A (ConA) at 100 gm/ml. The mol concentration of the glycolipid in the liposomes ranged from 5 to 14%, while

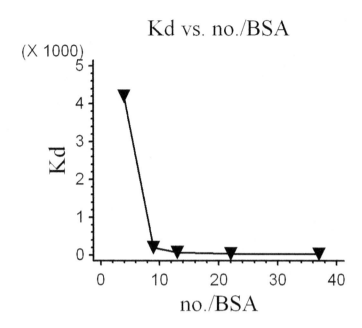

Fig. 8.3 Kd vs. no. glycan molecules per BSA site. The value drops precipitously from about 4,200 at $n=4$ to 194 at $n=9$, so that Kd is an order parameter that undergoes a change representing a topological transformation, here a cross-linking phase transition. A finer grain analysis would permit estimation of α in the relation 'Order Parameter' $\propto [(\rho - \rho_C)/\rho_C]^\alpha$ near the critical density ρ_C. Calculating an α from first principles would be a considerable scientific achievement.

the characteristic reaction duration – again, an order parameter – varied from 20.0 to 0.2 sec. with increasing concentration, as in Fig. 8.4.

   Orr *et al.* (1979) state:

> It is interesting to note that the lectin-induced aggregation ex-
> hibits a threshold or critical concentration effect. At incorporation
> levels of 5 mol % and less, the rate of the absorbance increase is slow,
> whereas at 7.5 mol % a dramatic increase in the rate is observed.

   In both experiments, finer grain observations would allow determination of α in the relation 'Order Parameter' $\propto [(\rho - \rho_C)/\rho_C]^\alpha$ near the critical area or volume density ρ_C. Calculating an α from first principles for different reacting chemical species would be a scientific tour de force.

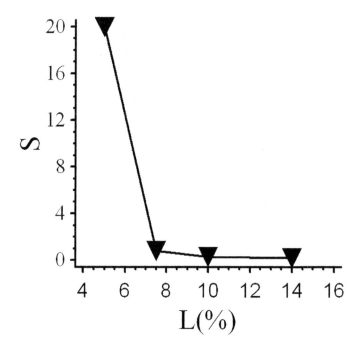

Fig. 8.4   Adapted from Orr *et al.* (1979). Critical concentration effect in aggregation of lecithin liposomes by fixed concentration of ConA. S, the inverse pseudo rate constant, is the order parameter that disappears at higher concentrations of lectin.

8.4   Information Catalysis

The basic idea

As noted above, information *per se* does not carry very much free energy, but the mechanisms that instantiate signals do, and this fact, in concert with the asymptotic limit theorems of information theory, permits an important evolutionary exaptation of entropic loss. Here, the essential index of interest may be density measures, but the argument seems more general.

Suppose there are two interacting information sources X, Y, emitting sequences of signals $x = [x_1, x_2, ...]$ and $y = [y_1, y_2, ...]$ at times $i = 1, 2, ...$ A joint sequence of signals $xy \equiv [(x_1, y_1), (x_2, y_2), ...]$ can then be defined, and, where the individual sequences x and y are correlated, it is possible to define a joint source information source uncertainty $H_{X,Y}$ for which a version of the information theory chain rule applies (Cover and Thomas, 2006):

$$H_{X,Y} < H_X + H_Y \, . \tag{8.3}$$

Again, one might expect the average production of information, $\hat{H}$, from a process having an available metabolic free energy rate M, to follow a relation of the form

$$\hat{H} = \frac{\int H \exp[-H/\kappa M] dH}{\int \exp[-H/\kappa M] dH} \approx \kappa M \, , \tag{8.4}$$

where κ is quite small, so the integral converges.

Then, from the chain rule,

$$\hat{H}_{X,Y} < \hat{H}_X + \hat{H}_Y \, ,$$
$$M_{X,Y} < M_X + M_Y \, . \tag{8.5}$$

If X is the system of interest, then, at the expense of maintaining the regulatory information source Y, it is possible to canalize the reaction paths of X: $M_{X,Y}$ becomes a valley in the larger energy structure created by imposing Y and X together. Thus high entropic loss – small κ – becomes a tool for regulating biochemical reactions.

A 'coevolutionary' model

In a now-familiar manner, again assume a larger set of interacting information sources, H_j, each associated with a free energy intensity M_j. Write each information source $\hat{H}_j \propto M_j$ as a function of a vector of 'density-like' parameters $\mathbf{K} = [K_1, K_2, ...]$.

For a simple physical system, one would expect a nonequilibrium thermodynamics driven by gradients in an entropy-like factor constructed from the $\hat{H}_j$ via analogs to empirical Onsager relations.

Define the usual set of 'information entropies' as the Legendre transforms

$$S_j \equiv \hat{H}_j - \sum_q K_q \partial \hat{H}_j / \partial K_q \propto$$
$$M_j - \sum_q K_q \partial M_j / \partial K_q \, . \tag{8.6}$$

Again, the simplest Onsager-like approach imposes dynamics driven by the gradients of the entropies as

$$dK_i/dt = \sum_j \mathcal{L}_{i,j} \partial S_j / \partial K_j \, . \tag{8.7}$$

where the $\mathcal{L}_{i,j}$ are empirical constants.

However, again following Champagnat *et al.* (2006), it is possible to take quite a different perspective, a 'coevolutionary' stochastic generalization in which the 'parameter vector' is the set of 'information' variates itself, $\mathbf{Q} = [\hat{H}_1, \hat{H}_2, ...] \propto [M_1, M_2, ...]$ rather than a set of external driving terms. That is, the M_j represent processes that drive each other and themselves in time. $\mathbf{Q}$ would, in turn, be constrained by a vector of channel capacities. Then, as in Champagnat *et al.*, the dynamical relations are given by phenomenological stochastic differential equations of the form

$$dQ_t^i = \mathcal{L}^i(t, \mathbf{Q})dt + \sum_j \sigma^{i,j}(t, \mathbf{Q})dB^j , \qquad (8.8)$$

or an analog using channel capacities. $\mathcal{L}$ and σ are appropriate functions and the dB represent stochastic 'noise' having characteristic quadratic variation (e.g., Protter, 1990).

These stochastic differential equations produce a coevolutionary – mutually driving – system so that setting them to to zero generates a collection of quasi-stable equilibria where transitions between them will be driven by 'large deviations' associated with yet other information sources: larger-scale, embedding, regulatory systems. The calculation is classic, and such large deviations can usually be represented by some entropy-like measure (e.g., Dembo and Zeitouni, 1998) that, in a biological context, is an embedding information source:

For Figs. 8.3 and 8.4, there are two such quasi-equilibria, described by the two phases indexed by collapse of the order parameters Kd and S, with experimenter-driven information – the systematic 'large deviation' of experimental changes in density measures – triggering the transition between them. These might be viewed as examples of biological logic gates, significantly larger, of course, than the more familiar neural synapse.

8.5   A Tiling Symmetry Model

A parallel perspective emerges by invoking an analog to the nonrigid molecule approach that Wallace (2011b, 2012b) has applied to intrinsically disordered proteins (IDP). Although we like to think of IDP and glycan/lectin reactions as in Fig. 8.1 in classical terms, invoking such metaphors as 'fly-casting', 'a snake slithering', 'glycan kelp bed' and so on, these are actually complicated processes of quantum chemistry – or some semiclassical approximation to it – that may benefit from more formal examination.

Longuet-Higgins (1963), in a classic paper, argues that:

The symmetry group of [a nonrigid] molecule is the set of (i) all feasible permutations of the positions and spins of identical nuclei and (ii) all feasible permutation-inversions, which simultaneously invert the coordinates of all particles in the centre of mass.

As for IDP (Wallace, 2011b, 2012b), assume it possible to extend non-rigid molecule group theory to 'kelp patches' of whip-like fronds anchored at one end, via wreath, semidirect, or other products over a set of finite and/or compact groups (e.g., Balasubramanian, 1980, 2004), or their groupoid generalizations, as now common in stereochemistry (Wallace, 2011c and cited references). These are taken as parameterized by an index of glycan 'topological complexity', in a large sense, a temperature-analog T which might simply be the number of exposed monosaccharides in the glycan kelp patch, the density of the kelp fronds, or some other such measure. In general, the number of group/groupoid elements can be expected to grow exponentially with T, typically as $\sum \Pi_j |G_j||A_j|^T$, where $|G_k|$ and $|A_k|$ are the size, in an appropriate sense, of symmetry groups G_k and A_k. See the Balasubramanian references for details.

Kahraman (2009) argues that the observed 'sloppiness' of large lock/small key molecular reaction dynamics suggests that binding site symmetry may be greater than binding ligand symmetries. Thus binding ligands may be expected to involve dual, mirror subgroups/groupoids of the anchored nonrigid group/groupoid symmetries of the glycan kelp patch. Thus the argument becomes:

Increasing $T, |G|, |A|$ → more flexibility → greatly enlarged binding site nonrigid symmetry group/groupoid → more subgroups/subtilings of possible binding sites for ligand attachment.

Glycan 'sequence flexibility', i.e., the way in which intrinsic glycan functions can be carried out by an ensemble of possible glycan structures, a continuum, mirrors, somewhat, the dynamic matching of the fuzzy-lock-and-key mechanisms suggested by Tompa and Fuxreiter (2008). Taking the approach of Wallace (2012b), this can be addressed by supposing that the duality between a subgroup/subgroupoid of the glycan frond patch and a set of binding ligands can be expressed as

$$\mathcal{B}_\alpha = C_\beta \mathcal{D}_\gamma \qquad (8.9)$$

where $\mathcal{B}_\alpha$ is a subgroup/groupoid (or set of them) of the glycan nonrigid symmetry group or groupoid, $\mathcal{D}_\gamma$ a similar structure of the set of binding ligands, and C_β is an appropriate inversion operation or set of them that represents static or dynamic matching between them. The fuzziness, however, now extends to sequence replacement as well as geometric variations, a far more complicated matter that may require an explicit extension of theory using groupoid methods and groupoid representations, as has been the case for stereochemistry (again, Wallace, 2011c and references). Groupoids are, in a sense, local symmetry structures that characterize the partial symmetries of finite tilings, quasicrystals, and the like.

An essential outcome of this approach is that the glycan/lectin patch matching symmetries, and their associated dynamics, should be highly punctuated in the parameter T that broadly indexes glycan topological complexity, for example the density effects of Figs. 8.3 and 8.4.

For large T, it becomes possible to apply a statistical mechanics analog, and to use Landau's spontaneous symmetry breaking/lifting approach via a Morse theory argument (Pettini, 2007). Typically, very many Morse functions are possible under a given circumstance, and we construct what is perhaps the simplest using group representations.

Taking an appropriate group representation in a particular matrix algebra, now construct a 'pseudo probability' $\mathcal{P}$ for nonrigid group element ω as

$$\mathcal{P}[\omega] = \frac{\exp[-|\chi_\omega|/\kappa T]}{\sum_\nu \exp[-|\chi_\nu|/\kappa T]}. \qquad (8.10)$$

χ_ϕ is the character of the group element ϕ in that representation, i.e., the trace of the matrix assigned to ϕ, and $|...|$ is the norm of the character, a real number. For systems that include compact groups, the sum may be a generalized integral.

The central idea is that F in the construct

$$\exp[-F/\kappa T] = \sum_\nu \exp[-|\chi_\nu|/\kappa T] \qquad (8.11)$$

is a Morse function in the topological temperature-analog T to which Landau's spontaneous symmetry breaking arguments apply (Pettini, 2007; Landau and Lifshitz, 2007), leading to the expectation of empirically observable highly punctuated structure and reaction dynamics in the index T that are the analog to phase transitions in 'simple' physical systems.

To reiterate, Landau's central insight was that, for many physical phenomena, raising the temperature would make accessible higher energy states of the system Hamiltonian, the quantum mechanical energy operator, and that the inherent symmetry changes would necessarily be punctuated. Here the focus is directly on a Morse function constructed from those symmetries, and the robustness of the underlying mathematics must carry through, basically an empirical question.

The basic assumption is that the group or groupoid tiling symmetries of the flexible glycan frond bed define the underlying lock that must be matched by an appropriate set of lectin keys, as in Fig. 8.1. Thus the statistical mechanics of glycan/lectin patch symmetries becomes central to reaction dynamics, according to an Onsager-like nonequilibrium thermodynamics formulation.

Define a 'symmetry entropy' based on the Morse function F of Eq. (8.11) over a set of underlying glycan structural or other parameters $\mathbf{Q} = [Q_1, ..., Q_n]$ as the Legendre transform

$$S = F(\mathbf{Q}) - \sum_i Q_i \partial F(\mathbf{Q})/\partial Q_i \,. \tag{8.12}$$

Again, the dynamics of such a system will be driven, at least in first approximation, by relations like Eq. (8.7):

$$dQ_i/dt = \sum_j \mathcal{K}_{i,j} \partial S/\partial Q_j \,, \tag{8.13}$$

where, again, the $\mathcal{K}_{i,j}$ are appropriate empirical parameters and t is the time.

Since, however, this is essentially a 'fuzzy' system, a more fitting approach is through a set of stochastic differential equations having the same form as Eq. (8.8):

$$dQ_t^i = \mathcal{K}_i(t, \mathbf{Q})dt + \sum_j \sigma_{i,j}(t, \mathbf{Q})dB^j \,, \tag{8.14}$$

where the $\mathcal{K}_i$ and $\sigma_{i,j}$ are appropriate functions.

Again, different kinds of 'noise' dB^j will have particular forms of quadratic variation affecting dynamics.

Setting this equation to zero and solving for stationary points gives attractor states, since, again, noise precludes unstable equilibria, although the solution may, in fact, be a highly dynamic strange attractor set.

The essential point here is that setting Eq. (8.14) to zero again directly generates an index theorem (Hazewinkel, 2002) in the sense of Atiyah and Singer (1963) that relates analytic results – the solutions of the equations – to an underlying set of topological structures representing the eigenmodes of a complicated 'nonrigid molecule' geometric operator whose group/groupoid spectrum represents the symmetries of the possible glycan kelp patch lock/lectin key set reactions that must take place for information to be transmitted, i.e., for the chemical logic gate to be triggered.

8.6 Summary

For even a 'simple' renormalization model of glycan/lectin reaction phase transitions, the 'universality' exponent α, following the arguments of the Mathematical Appendix, is unlikely to be universal, and indeed should be a precisely distinguishing characteristic of both the reacting species and the modes of their reactions. Thus, the 'failure' of universality might well be a tool that allows insight into the energy landscapes of $M_{X,Y}$, M_X and M_Y, the resulting canalization via information catalysis, and its 'coevolutionary' correlates. Indeed, biology is not physics, and, typically, evolution may exapt, in the sense of Gould (2002), mechanisms that can distinguish reacting chemical species and/or their modes of reaction.

Underlying the general approach is a biological version of the spontaneous symmetry change perspective so popular in current physical theory. The symmetries, however, may not be as 'pure' as those most familiar to physicists and, as described, might involve such complexities as nonrigid molecule groupoid tilings and their wreath products. Nonetheless, the line of argument implied by Figs. 8.1 and 8.3 is quite compelling, and the techniques of the Mathematical Appendix may aid in the calculation of spectra of 'universality' constants for such experiments from first principles.

What becomes obvious, almost in passing, is the utterly central point that the *in vitro* glycan/lectin phase transitions characterized by Figs. 8.3 and 8.4 imply the operation of complicated biological logic gates *in vivo* that must be nearly as sophisticated as the more familiar neural synaptic switches, if on different scales. Cascades of even 'simple' logic gates can carry out very complex computational processes, and these arguments add yet further weight to a perspective that sees the living state as characterized by cognitive phenomena at virtually every scale and level of organization – the biological cognome.

Chapter 9

EXAMPLE: IDP LOGIC GATES

9.1   Introduction

Tompa *et al.* (2005) have observed that intrinsically disordered proteins provide unprecedented examples of protein signal moonlighting – multiple, often unrelated, functions of the same molecule – by eliciting both inhibiting and activating action on different partners, or even on the same partner. Figure 9.1, adapted from their paper, provides one schematic. The disordered protein can bind to more than one site on the partner molecule represented by a tilted square on the left of the figure. Binding to one site, as indicated by the shaded oval, creates an activated conformation, while binding to another site, the rectangle, results in an inhibited complex. Tompa *et al.* (2005) indicate several different such possible mechanisms that are not mutually exclusive, but we will focus on this particular example. Generalization is direct.

Wallace (2012b) has described IDP reaction dynamics via a statistical mechanics approach to a 'symmetry spectrum' derived from a groupoid generalization of the wreath product of groups (e.g., Houghton, 1975) that characterizes 'conventional' nonrigid molecule theory (e.g., Longuet-Higgins, 1963; Balasubramanian, 1980). The essential point is that the 'fuzzy lock-and-key' involves matching subgroups/subgroupoids between IDP and binding ligand via a set of mirror symmetries. The number of group/groupoid elements in a wreath product, related to the number of possible subgroups/subgroupoids, typically grows as the exponential power of the number of amino acids making up the IDP. That is, long IDPs have exponentially more possible linkages like that of Fig. 9.1 than do short.

More complete discussions of IDP from different perspectives can be found in Uversky (2002) and Jeffery (2005).

Activated conformation

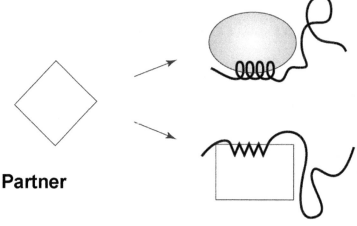

Partner

Inhibited conformation

Fig. 9.1 Adapted from Tompa *et al.* (2005). The partner, represented by the tilted square, can bind in two ways with the incoming IDP. The shaded oval represents activated, and the rectangle, inhibited species. The 'choice' between them is, in this model, to be made by an information catalysis in which an incoming signal shifts the lowest energy state between the two otherwise thermodynamically competitive conformations. This is one example of a vast spectrum of similar chemical 'logic gates'.

For generalized switches and logic gates like Fig. 9.1, however, a comprehensive approach is necessary that reflects the operation of an elaborate regulatory system of chemical cognition analogous to what has been used to describe the immune system (Atlan and Cohen, 1998; Cohen, 2000) or higher order neural and social function (e.g., Wallace, 2005; Wallace and Fullilove, 2008).

This overall idea has, in fact, been a subject of both speculation and research since the late 1930s, and is not restricted to intrinsically disordered proteins. There are many current and past examples, following the excellent review of James and Tawfik (2003). The essential point is that a single protein may equilibrate between thermodynamically equivalent preexisting conformations until one is 'chosen', in a sense, by some external signal:

1. Volkman *et al.* (2001) show that the protein NtrC is allostatically regulated by phosphorylation. Two conformations are present in unphosphorylated NtrC, with phosphorylation merely shifting the equilibrium toward the active conformation.

2. Cordes *et al.* (2000) show that, with regard to the DNA-binding domain of the Arc repressor, the Arc-N11L mutant spontaneously interconverts between a two-stranded antiparallel β sheet and a two-3_{10}-helix structure. In the absence of a DNA ligand, the two conformations are in equilibrium at almost equal proportions. Addition of the DNA ligand shifts the equilibrium towards the β-sheet form.

3. According to Chien and Weissman (2001), the prion protein PrP interconverts between an α-helix PrP^c and an all β-sheet conformation PrP^{sc}. The β-sheet is trapped by subsequent oligomerization, resulting in amyloid deposit and the onset of disease.

4. Very early on, Pauling (1940) and Landsteiner (1936) proposed that some proteins – antibodies – can exist as an ensemble of isomers with different structures but with similar free energy, so that, if each isomer was able to bind to a different ligand, functional diversity could go far beyond sequence diversity.

The usual formal development, based on the immune system example, leads to the idea of cognitive control in moonlighting pleiotropy, and by inference, for many other 'logic gate' structures as well. To reiterate, from the perspective of Atlan and Cohen (1998), who introduce a cognitive paradigm for the immune system, cognition involves comparison of a perceived signal with an internal, learned or inherited, picture of the world, and, upon that comparison, choice of a single response from a larger repertoire of possible responses. This inherently involves the transmission of information, since choice always necessitates a reduction in uncertainty (e.g., Ash, 1990, p. 21).

'Cognition', in that sense, is quite routine, since even a thermostat would be cognitive from this perspective. The essential point is that sufficiently large biological structures can follow a great multiplicity of possible isoenergetic 'reaction paths', and focus must thereupon shift from the details of the chemical machinery itself to the details of its behavior in the context of signals, moving from what the system is in terms of its detailed molecular structure, to examining what it does. In computer terminology, this is analogous to focusing on the program the machine carries out rather than on a detailed study of the state of each logic gate at each clock cycle.

9.2   Symbolic Dynamics of Molecular Switching

Symbolic dynamics is a coarse-grained perspective on dynamic structures and processes that discretizes their time trajectories in terms of accessible regions so that it is possible to do statistical mechanics on symbol sequences (e.g., McCauley, 1993, Ch. 8) that can be said to constitute an 'alphabet'. Within that 'alphabet', certain 'statements' are highly probable, and others far less so.

To reiterate something of Chapter 4, the simple (ideal) oscillating reaction described by the equations

$$dX/dt = \omega Y, dY/dt = -\omega X$$

has the solution

$$X(t) = \sin(\omega t), Y(t) = \cos(\omega t)$$

so that

$$X(t)^2 + Y(t)^2 \equiv 1,$$

and the system traces out an endless circular trajectory in time. Divide the $X - Y$ plane into two components, the simplest possible coarse-graining, calling the halfplane to the left of the vertical Y axis A and that to the right B. This system, over units of the period $1/(2\pi\omega)$, traces out a stream of As and Bs having a very precise grammar and syntax: ABABABAB...

Again, many other such statements might be conceivable, e.g., AAAAAA..., BBBBB..., AAABAAAB..., ABAABAAAB..., and so on, but, of the infinite number of possibilities, there is only one actually observed, that is 'grammatical'.

More complex dynamical reaction models, incorporating diffusional drift around deterministic solutions, or elaborate structures of complicated stochastic differential equations having various domains of attraction – different sets of 'grammars' – can be described by analogous means (e.g., Beck and Schlogl, 1995, Ch. 3).

Again, following Section 4.2, rather than taking symbolic dynamics as a simplification of more exact analytic or stochastic approaches, it is possible to comprehensively generalize the technique itself. Complicated cellular processes may not have identifiable sets of stochastic differential equations like noisy, nonlinear mechanical clocks, but, under appropriate coarse-graining, they may still have recognizable sets of grammar and syntax over the long term. Proper coarse-graining may, however, often be the hard scientific problem.

The fundamental assumption for complicated biological reactions like the change in function between the upper and lower complexes of Fig. 9.1 is that reaction trajectories can be classified into two groups, a very large set that has essentially zero probability, and a much smaller 'grammatical' set. For the grammatical/syntactical set, the argument is – again – that, given a set of elaborate trajectories of length n, the number of grammatical ones, $N(n)$, follows a limit law of the form

$$H = \lim_{n \to \infty} \frac{\log[N(n)]}{n} \tag{9.1}$$

such that H both exists and is independent of path. If convergence occurs for some finite n_H, then the process is said to be of order n_H. This is a critical foundation of, and limitation on, the modeling strategy adopted here, and constrains its possible realm of applicability. It is, however, fairly general in that it is independent of the serial correlations along reaction pathways.

The basic idea is shown in Fig. 9.2, where an initial IDP/partner configuration, $\mathbf{S}_0$, can either converge on an activated IDP complex $\mathbf{S}_{act}$ via the set of high probability reaction paths to the left of the filled triangle, or it can converge to a thermodynamically competitive inhibited state $\mathbf{S}_{inhib}$ to the right.

The approach, via coarse-graining and symbolic dynamics, assigns classic information sources to the two sets of thermodynamically competitive 'grammatical' pathways. The essential question is how a regulatory catalysis can act in such a circumstance to change the probabilities of convergence on $\mathbf{S}_{act}$ or $\mathbf{S}_{inhib}$.

9.3 Another Dual Information Source

The first step in answering that question lies in describing the activity of a large class of regulatory activity in terms of another information source.

Formally, and by now, familiarly, a pattern of incoming input $\mathbf{S}_i$ describing the status of the IDP/partner configuration – starting with the initial state $\mathbf{S}_0$ – is mixed in a systematic algorithmic manner with a pattern of otherwise unspecified 'ongoing activity', including cellular, epigenetic and environmental signals, $\mathbf{W}_i$, to create a path of combined signals $x = (a_0, a_1, ..., a_n, ...)$. Each a_k thus represents some functional composition of internal and external factors, and is expressed in terms of the

Sact
Sinhib

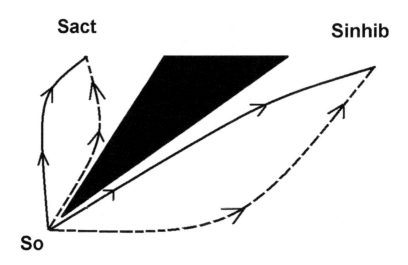

So

Fig. 9.2 An initial IDP/partner configuration $\mathbf{S}_0$ can either converge on an active final configuration $\mathbf{S}_{act}$ via the set of high probability reaction paths to the left of the filled triangle, or it can converge to a thermodynamically competitive inhibited state $\mathbf{S}_{inhib}$ to the right.

intermediate states as

$$\mathbf{S}_{i+1} = f([\mathbf{S}_i, \mathbf{W}_i]) = f(a_i) \qquad (9.2)$$

for some unspecified function f. The a_i are seen to be very complicated composite objects, in this treatment, that we may choose to coarse-grain so as to obtain an appropriate 'alphabet'.

Most simply, $\mathbf{S}$ would be a vector, $\mathbf{W}$ a matrix, and f would be a function of their product at 'time' i.

To reiterate earlier arguments, the path x is fed into a highly nonlinear decision function, h, a sudden threshold pattern recognition structure, in a sense, that generates an output $h(x)$ that is an element of one of two disjoint sets B_0 and B_1 of possible system responses. Again, define the sets B_k as $B_0 = \{b_0, ..., b_k\}, B_1 = \{b_{k+1}, ..., b_m\}$.

As in the earlier chapters, assume an elaborate graded response, in precisely the sense studied by Pufall *et al.* (2005), supposing that if $h(x) \in B_0$, the pattern is not recognized, and if $h(x) \in B_1$, the pattern has been recognized, and some action $b_j, k + 1 \leq j \leq m$ takes place. Typically, for the example of Fig. 9.2, the set B_1 would represent the final state of the IDP/final partner complex, either activated or inhibited, that is sent on in the sequence of biological processes.

Again, the principal objects of formal interest are paths x triggering pattern recognition and response. That is, given a fixed initial state $a_0 = [\mathbf{S}_0, \mathbf{W}_0]$, examine all possible subsequent paths x beginning with a_0 and leading to the event $h(x) \in B_1$. Thus $h(a_0, ..., a_j) \in B_0$ for all $0 < j < m$, but $h(a_0, ..., a_m) \in B_1$. B_1 is thus the set of final possible states, $\{\mathbf{S}_{act}\} \cup \{\mathbf{S}_{inhib}\}$ from Fig. 9.2 that includes both the active and inhibited complexes.

Again, for each positive integer n, let $N(n)$ be the number of high probability grammatical and syntactical paths of length n which begin with some particular a_0 and lead to the condition $h(x) \in B_1$. Call such paths 'meaningful', assuming that $N(n)$ will be considerably less than the number of all possible paths of length n leading from a_0 to the condition $h(x) \in B_1$.

Again, while the combining algorithm, the form of the nonlinear oscillator, and the details of grammar and syntax, can all be unspecified in this model, the critical assumption that permits inference of the necessary conditions constrained by the asymptotic limit theorems of information theory is that, again, the finite limit $H = \lim_{n\to\infty} \log[N(n)]/n$ both exists and is independent of the path x.

Recall that not all cognitive processes are likely to be ergodic in this sense, implying that H, if it indeed exists at all, is path dependent, although extension to nearly ergodic processes seems possible (e.g., Wallace and Fullilove, 2008).

Again, invoking the spirit of the Shannon–McMillan theorem, as choice involves an inherent reduction in uncertainty, it is then possible to define an adiabatically, piecewise stationary, ergodic (APSE) information source $\mathbf{X}$ associated with stochastic variates X_j having joint and conditional probabilities $P(a_0, ..., a_n)$ and $P(a_n|a_0, ..., a_{n-1})$ such that appropriate conditional and joint Shannon uncertainties satisfy the classic information theory relations of Eq. (1.2).

This is, again, the dual information source to the underlying ergodic cognitive process.

9.4 Information Catalysis

In the limit of large n, $H = \lim_{n\to\infty} \log[N(n)]/n$ becomes homologous to the free energy density of a physical system at the thermodynamic limit of infinite volume.

Information catalysis, in the circumstance of Fig. 9.2, again arises most simply via the information theory chain rule (Cover and Thomas, 2006). Given X as the information source representing the reaction paths of Fig. 9.2, and Y, an information source dual to the sophisticated chemical cognition of the regulating system, one can define jointly typical paths $z_i = (x_i, y_i)$ having the joint information source uncertainty $H(X, Y)$ satisfying the standard relation $H(X, Y) = H(X) + H(Y|X) \leq H(X) + H(Y)$.

Of necessity, by the arguments of Section 2.3, within a cell, there will be an ensemble of possible reactions, driven by available metabolic free energy, so that, taking $< .. >$ as representing an average, $[< H(X, Y) >] < [< H(X) > + < H(Y) >]$.

Again, letting M represent the intensity of available metabolic free energy,

$$< H >= \frac{\int H \exp[-H/\kappa M]dH}{\int \exp[-H/\kappa M]dH} \approx \kappa M,$$

where κ, an inverse energy intensity scaling constant, may be quite small indeed, a consequence of entropic translation losses between metabolic free energy and the expression of information.

The resulting expression, $M_{X,Y} < M_X + M_Y$, again suggests an explicit free energy mechanism for reaction canalization. Something much like the arguments of Section 8.5 seems applicable here as well.

9.5 Summary

Wallace (2012b), using a groupoid extension of conventional nonrigid molecule theory, introduced a literally astronomically large spectrum of possible symmetry classifications for IDP/partner complexes. The size of the appropriate symmetry group (or groupoid) must grow exponentially in the number of amino acid bases within the flexible IDP frond. For 30 to 100 amino acids, the nonrigid symmetry set is indeed astronomical, and can only be addressed by a statistical mechanics argument.

The particular utility of IDPs for moonlighting, as inferred from Tompa *et al.* (2005), appears possible through the massive number of subgroup/tiling mirror image matchings that are available to the molecular fuzzy lock-and-key, as governed by a regulatory structure that is likely to be another example of sophisticated chemical cognition, akin to the immune system. Given these results, cognitive biochemical processes regulating IDP moonlighting are not likely to yield to exact 'chemical' description, not only from considerations of IDP symmetry group magnitude, but because their dynamics are particularly contingent on other signals that may arise from higher level, embedding, cognitive regulatory processes.

However, such behaviors, in terms of the dual information source, are nonetheless constrained by the asymptotic limit theorems of information theory, and this may allow construction of regression model-like statistical tools useful for scientific inference, focusing on the behaviors of the system rather than on a detailed description of its mechanical state under all circumstances and at all times. Again, the analogy is to describe the behavior of a computer in terms of its program, rather than attempting to provide a full cross-sectional description of the state of each logic gate at each clock cycle.

It should be particularly emphasized that many of the composite of IDP–partner–regulator 'logic gates' in Fig. 1 of Tompa *et al.* (2005) are likely to be quite different from 'simple' computer models, having extraordinarily subtle properties. There is no reason to believe evolution is restricted to binary mathematics (AND, OR, XOR, etc.). For example, Kung *et al.* (2012), in their description of 'molecular juggling' in B_{12} complexes, write:

> B_{12}-dependent methyl transfer lies at the heart of methylation biochemistry and is an essential [biological] reaction... Overall, our data indicate that B_{12} domain movement is not a simple, two-state switch between 'resting' and 'catalytic' conformations. Instead, a flexible B_{12} domain samples an ensemble of conformations, where subtle shifts of the conformational equilibrium place B_{12} progressively closer to the active site, thereby increasing the population of conformers capable of methyl transfer without obstructing substrate access or hindering domain movement.

Much of what we conjecture here is already common currency within protein science, although not, perhaps, systematized into a consistent mathematical formalism. Almost all the proposed mechanisms have been described using a different vocabulary, and, taking the suggestion of a commentator, the following table attempts a translation of the model.

Model Term	Protein Science Term
Subgroup/subgroupoid	Protein conformation
Cognition	Molecular recognition
Subgroup tiling	Conformation selection
Internal picture of the world	Preformed structural elements
Information catalysis	Cooperative structure transition

Finally, these considerations add further weight to the perspective that sees a fundamental defining characteristic of the living state as the operation of cognitive processes at virtually all scales and levels of organization: the foundation of the human cognome, as presented here.

Chapter 10

TREATMENT

How is the system of nested cognitive processes that constitute the human cognome to be brought back to normal function when it suffers pathological change? The multilevel, multiscale characteristics explored in the previous chapters suggest the necessity of similarly complicated – indeed, mirror image – interventions that act across scale and level of organization. Models of treatment and treatment failure are then, by necessity, ultimately as complicated as the cognome network itself. This inherent complexity is mitigated, however, by a 'small world' structure of that network that greatly enhances the centrality of culture, historical trajectory, social relations, and institutional form and behavior.

Figure 1.1 implies we have run out of magic bullets, but the possibility of magic strategies remains. It will become clear, however, that therapeutic alteration of the cognome faces the same pitfall of programming and stability that bedevils coevolutionary computing systems, recognized here as 'side effects' (Wallace, 2009b, 2010b).

10.1 The Generalized Retina

Cohen (2000) argues for an 'immunological homunculus' as the immune system's perception of the body as a whole. The particular utility of such a thing, in his view, is that sensing perturbations in a bodily self-image can serve as an early warning sign of pending necessary inflammatory response – expressions of tumorigenesis, acute or chronic infection, parasitization, and the like. Thayer and Lane (2000) argue something analogous for emotional response as a quick internal index of larger patterns of threat or opportunity.

It seems obvious that the tunable, shifting global broadcasts of interacting cognitive submodules explored above must also have coherent internal self-images of the states of the mind/body and its social relationships. Such an inferred picture might be termed a 'generalized retina' (GR). It is possible to use the responses of the GR to characterize physiological/mental responses to both illness and to medical interventions used to treat that illness. Illness and treatment may then come to reflect one another in a hall of mirrors reminiscent of Jerne's idiotypic network proposed for the dynamics of the immune system. The inevitable canonical and idiosyncratic instabilities of coevolutionary/idiotypic systems then become manifest as side effects.

Suppose, rather than measuring either stress or cognitive submodule and broadcast function directly, it is possible to determine the concentrations of hormones, neurotransmitters, certain cytokines, and other biomarkers, or else macroscopic behaviors, beliefs, feelings, or other responses associated with the function of cognitive submodules according to some natural time frame inherent to the system. This would typically be the circadian cycle in both men and women, and the hormonal cycle in premenopausal women. Suppose, in the absence of extraordinary meaningful psychosocial stress, it is possible to measure a series of n biomarker concentrations, behavioral characteristics, and other indices at time t which we represent as an n-dimensional vector X_t. Suppose it possible to conduct a number of experiments, and create a regression model so that, in the absence of perturbation, it becomes possible to write, to first order, the set of markers at time $t + 1$ in terms of that at time t using a matrix equation of the form

$$X_{t+1} \approx \mathbf{R}X_t, \tag{10.1}$$

where $\mathbf{R}$ is the matrix of regression coefficients, with normalization to a zero vector of constant terms.

Write a GR response to short-term perturbation as

$$X_{t+1} = (\mathbf{R}_0 + \delta\mathbf{R}_{t+1})X_t,$$

where $\delta\mathbf{R}$ represents variation of the generalized cognitive self-image about the basic state $\mathbf{R}_0$.

Now impose a Jordan block diagonalization in terms of the matrix of (generally nonorthogonal) eigenvectors $\mathbf{Q}_0$ of some 'zero reference state' $\mathbf{R}_0$, obtaining, for an initial condition that is an eigenvector $Y_t \equiv Y_k$ of $\mathbf{J}_0 = \mathbf{Q}_0\mathbf{R}_0\mathbf{Q}_0^{-1}$,

$$Y_{t+1} = (\mathbf{J}_0 + \delta\mathbf{J}_{t+1})Y_k = \lambda_k Y_k + \delta Y_{t+1} =$$

$$\lambda_k Y_k + \sum_{j=1}^{n} a_j Y_j, \tag{10.2}$$

where $\mathbf{J}_0$ is a (block) diagonal matrix as above, $\delta\mathbf{J}_{t+1} \equiv \mathbf{Q}_0\delta\mathbf{R}_{t+1}\mathbf{Q}_0^{-1}$, and δY_{t+1} *has been expanded in terms of a spectrum of the eigenvectors of* $\mathbf{J}_0$, with

$$|a_j| \ll |\lambda_k|, |a_{j+1}| \ll |a_j|. \tag{10.3}$$

The essential point is that, provided $\mathbf{R}_0$ has been properly tuned, so that this condition is true, the first few terms in the spectrum of the pleiotropic iteration of the eigenstate will contain almost all of the essential information about the perturbation, i.e., most of the variance. This is precisely similar to the detection of color in the optical retina, where three overlapping non-orthogonal 'eigenmodes' of response suffice to characterize a vast array of color sensations. Here, if a concise spectral expansion is possible, a very small number of (typically nonorthogonal) 'generalized cognitive eigenmodes' permit characterization of a vast range of external perturbations, and rate distortion constraints become very manageable indeed. Thus, GR responses – the spectrum of excited eigenmodes of $\mathbf{R}_0$, provided it is properly tuned – can be a very accurate and precise gage of environmental perturbation.

The choice of zero reference state $\mathbf{R}_0$, the 'base state' from which perturbations are measured, is, apparently, a highly nontrivial task, necessitating a specialized apparatus.

This is no small matter. According to current theory, the adapted human mind functions through the action and interaction of distinct mental modules that evolved fairly rapidly to help address special problems of environmental and social selection pressure faced by our Pleistocene ancestors (Barkow *et al.*, 1992). It appears necessary to postulate many other interacting physiological and social cognitive modules – the human cognome. As is well known in computer engineering, calculation by specialized submodules – numeric processor chips – can be a far more efficient means of solving particular well-defined classes of problems than direct computation by a generalized system. It appears, then, that generalized physiological cognition has evolved specialized submodules to speed the address of certain commonly recurring challenges. Nunney (1999) has argued that, as a power law of cell count, specialized subsystems are increasingly required to recognize and redress tumorigenesis, mechanisms ranging from molecular error-correcting codes, to programmed cell death, and finally full-blown immune attack.

It seems that identification of the designated normal state of the GR – generalized cognition's self-image of the body and its social relationships –

is difficult, requiring a dedicated cognitive submodule within overall generalized cognition. This is essentially because, for the vast majority of information systems, unlike mechanical systems, there are no restoring springs whose low energy state automatically identifies equilibrium: relatively speaking, all states of the GR are 'high energy' states, particularly in view of the massive entropic losses associated with the physical instantiation of information. That is, active comparison must be made of the state of the GR with some stored internal reference picture, and a decision made about whether to reset to zero, which is a cognitive process. The complexity of such a submodule may also follow something like Nunney's power law with animal size, as the overall generalized cognition and its image of the self, become increasingly complicated with rising number of cells and levels of linked cognition.

Failure of that cognitive submodule can result in identification of an excited state of the GR as normal, triggering the collective patterns of systemic activation that, following the argument of Wallace (2004), constitute certain comorbid mental and chronic physical disorders. This would result in a relatively small number of characteristic eigenforms of comorbidity, which would typically become more mixed with increasing disorder.

In sum, since such 'zero mode identification' (ZMI) is a (presumed) cognitive submodule of overall generalized cognition, it involves convoluting incoming 'sensory' with 'ongoing' internal memory data in choosing the zero state, i.e., defining $\mathbf{R}_0$. The dual information source defined by this cognitive process can then interact in a punctuated manner with 'external information sources' according to the rate distortion and related arguments above. From a rate distortion theorem perspective, then, those external information sources literally write a distorted image of themselves onto the ZMI, often in a punctuated manner: (relatively) sudden onset of a developmental trajectory to comorbid mental disorders and pathophysiology.

Different systems of external signals – including but not limited to structured psychosocial stress – will, presumably, write different characteristic images of themselves onto the ZMI cognitive submodule, i.e., trigger different eigenpatterns of comorbid mental/physical disorder.

A brief reformulation in abstract terms may be of interest. Recall that the essential characteristic of cognition in this formalism involves a function h which maps a (convolutional) path $x = a_0, a_1, ..., a_n, ...$ onto a member of one of two disjoint sets, B_0 or B_1. Thus, respectively, either (1) $h(x) \in B_0$, implying no action taken, or, (2) $h(x) \in B_1$, and some particular response is chosen from a large repertoire of possible responses. Some 'higher order cognitive module' might be needed to identify what constituted B_0, the set of 'normal' states. Again, this is because that, for information systems, virtually all states are more or less isoenergetic, and there is no way to identify a ground state using the physicist's favorite variational or other minimization arguments on energy, in the absence of an embedding 'information catalyst'.

Suppose that higher order cognitive module, now recognizable as precisely such a catalyst, interacts with an embedding language of structured psychosocial stress (or other systemic perturbation) and, instantiating a rate distortion image of that embedding stress, begins to include one or more members of the set B_1 into the set B_0. Recurrent 'hits' on that aberrant state would be experienced as episodes of highly structured comorbid mind/body pathology.

Empirical tests of this hypothesis, however, quickly lead again into real-world regression models involving the interrelations of measurable biomarkers, beliefs, behaviors, feelings, and so on, requiring formalism much like that used above. The GR can, then, be viewed as a generic heuristic device typifying such regression approaches.

The generalized retina is more appropriately characterized as a 'rate distortion manifold', a local projection that, through overlap, has global structure, much like the tangent planes to a complicated geometric object. Glazebrook and Wallace (2009a) provide more detailed mathematical treatment. Some thought will show that the GR and the more abstract rate distortion manifold are explicit examples of the general tuning theorem argument of the Mathematical Appendix that is a version of the 'no free lunch' restriction described in Section 2.1.

10.2 Therapeutic Efficacy

To reiterate, if $\mathbf{X}$ represents the information source dual to the 'zero mode identification' information catalyst in a generalized cognition, and if $\mathbf{Z}$ is the information source characterizing structured psychosocial stress or other noxious embedding context, the mutual information between them

$$I(\mathbf{X}; \mathbf{Z}) = H(\mathbf{X}) - H(\mathbf{X}|\mathbf{Z}) \qquad (10.4)$$

serves as a splitting criterion for pairs of linked paths of states.

Suppose it possible to parameterize the coupling between these interacting information sources by some appropriate index, ω, writing

$$I(\mathbf{X}; \mathbf{Z}) = I[\omega] \,, \tag{10.5}$$

with structured psychosocial stress or some other noxious condition as the embedding context.

Socioculturally constructed and structured psychosocial stress or other noxious exposure, in this model having both (generalized) grammar and syntax, can be viewed as entraining the function of zero mode identification when the coupling with stress exceeds a threshold, following the arguments of Section 2.2.

More than one threshold appears likely, accounting, in a sense, for the typically staged nature of environmentally caused disorders. These should result in a synergistic – i.e., comorbidly excited – mixed affective, rationally cognitive, psychosocial, and inflammatory or other physical excited state of otherwise normal response. This excited state is the effect of stress on the linked decision processes of various cognitive functions, in particular, acting through the identification of a false 'zero mode' of the GR. This is a collective, but highly systematic, 'tuning failure' that, in the rate distortion sense, constitutes a literal image of the structure of imposed pathogenic context written upon the ability of the GR to characterize a normal condition of excitation, causing a mixed, shifting, highly dynamic excited state of chronically comorbid mental and physical disorder.

In this model, different eigenmodes Y_k of the GR regression model characterized by the matrix $\mathbf{R}_0$ can be taken as the 'shifting-of-gears' between different 'languages' defining the sets B_0 and B_1. That is, different eigenmodes of the GR would correspond to different required (and possibly mixed) highly dynamic characteristic systemic responses.

If there is a state (or set of states) Y_1 such that $\mathbf{R}_0 Y_1 = Y_1$, then the 'unitary kernel' Y_1 corresponds to the condition 'no response required', the set B_0.

Suppose pathology becomes manifest,

$$\mathbf{R}_0 \to \mathbf{R}_0 + \delta \mathbf{R} \equiv \hat{\mathbf{R}}_0,$$

so that, for example, some chronic excited state becomes the new 'unitary kernel', and

$$Y_1 \to \hat{Y}_1 \neq Y_1$$

$$\hat{\mathbf{R}}_0 \hat{Y}_1 = \hat{Y}_1.$$

This could be chronic inflammation, autoimmune response, persistent depression/anxiety or HPA axis activation/burnout, and so on.

Medical intervention – a kind of reprogramming of a highly coevolutionary/idiotypic cognitive system – seeks to induce a sequence of therapeutic counterperturbations $\delta \mathbf{T}_k$ according to the pattern:

$$\begin{aligned}
&[\hat{\mathbf{R}}_0 + \delta \mathbf{T}_1]\hat{Y}_1 = Y^1\,, \\
&\hat{\mathbf{R}}_1 \equiv \hat{\mathbf{R}}_0 + \delta \mathbf{T}_1\,, \\
&[\hat{\mathbf{R}}_1 + \delta \mathbf{T}_2]Y^1 = Y^2\,, \\
&\cdots
\end{aligned} \tag{10.6}$$

and so on, such that, using an appropriate metric,

$$Y^j \to Y_1\,. \tag{10.7}$$

That is, the multilevel, highly dynamic, shifting, tunable system of global broadcasts – the mind/body system of the cognome – as monitored by the GR, is driven to its original condition.

The condition $\hat{\mathbf{R}}_0 \to \mathbf{R}_0$ may or may not be met. That is, actual cure may not be possible, in which case palliation or control is the therapeutic aim, involving persistent application of therapeutic perturbations $\delta \mathbf{T}_j$.

The essential point is that the pathological state $\hat{\mathbf{R}}_0$ and the sequence of inherently multiscale therapeutic interventions $\delta \mathbf{T}_k, k = 1, 2, \ldots$ are interactive and reflective, depending on the regression of the set of vectors Y^j to the desired state Y_1, much in the same spirit as Jerne's immunological idiotypic hall of mirrors.

The therapeutic problem revolves around minimizing the difference between Y^k and Y_1 over the course of treatment: that difference is the inextricable convolution of 'treatment failure' with 'adverse reactions' to the course of treatment itself, and 'failure of compliance' attributed through social construction by provider to patient, i.e., failure of the therapeutic alliance, in the sense of Brock and Salinsky (1993).

It should be obvious that the treatment sequence $\delta \mathbf{T}_k$ is itself a cognitive path of interventions having, in turn, a dual information source in the sense previously invoked.

Treatment may, then, interact in the usual rate distortion manner with patterns of structured pathogenic context that are, themselves, signals from an embedding information source. Thus, treatment failure, adverse reactions, and patient noncompliance will, of necessity, embody a distorted image of that context.

In sum, characteristic patterns of treatment failure, adverse reactions, and patient noncompliance reflecting collapse of the therapeutic alliance, will occur in virtually all therapeutic interventions – even those acting across scale – according to the manner in which structured psychosocial stress or other embedding noxious conditions are expressed as an image within the multiscale treatment process. This would most likely occur in a highly punctuated manner, depending in a quantitative way on the degree of coupling of the threefold system of affected individual, patient/provider interaction, and multilevel treatment mode, with that stress or condition.

Given that the principal environment of humans is defined by interaction with other humans and their socioeconomic institutions, social effects, in particular, are likely to be dominant, and we now explore this in more detail.

10.3   Psychosocial Stress

Stress, in human populations, is not a random sequence of perturbations, and is not independent of its perception. Rather, it involves a highly correlated, grammatical, syntactical process by which an embedding psychosocial environment communicates with an individual, particularly with that individual's HPA axis, in the context of social hierarchy. Thus, the stress experienced by an individual can, in first approximation, be viewed as an adiabatically piecewise stationary ergodic (APSE) information source, interacting with a similar dual information source defined by HPA axis cognition, in the sense of Chapter 1.

The ergodic nature of the 'language' of stress – its essential characteristic as an information source – is a generalization of the law of large numbers, so that long-time averages can be well approximated by cross-sectional expectations. Languages do not have simple autocorrelation patterns, in distinct contrast with the usual assumption of random perturbations by white noise in the standard formulation of stochastic differential equations.

To quantitatively measure stress, determine the concentrations of HPA axis hormones and other biomarkers according to some natural time frame, the inherent period of the system. In the absence of extraordinary meaningful psychosocial stress, measure a series of n concentrations at time t, represented as an n-dimensional vector X_t. Conduct a number of such experiments, and create a regression model that can, in the absence of perturbation, write, to first order, the concentration of biomarkers at time $t+1$ in terms of that at time t using the matrix equation

$$X_{t+1} \approx < \mathbf{U} > X_t + b_0 . \tag{10.8}$$

$< \mathbf{U} >$ is the matrix of regression coefficients and b_0 a vector of constant terms.

Suppose, in the presence of a perturbation by structured stress,

$$X_{t+1} = (< \mathbf{U} > +\delta \mathbf{U}_{t+1})X_t + b_0 \equiv < \mathbf{U} > X_t + \epsilon_{t+1}, \qquad (10.9)$$

where both b_0 and $\delta \mathbf{U}_{t+1}X_t$ have been absorbed into a vector ϵ_{t+1} of error terms that are not necessarily small in this formulation.

It is important to realize that this is not a population process whose continuous analog is exponential growth. Rather, it is more akin to the passage of a signal – structured psychosocial stress – through a distorting physiological filter.

If the matrix of regression coefficients $< \mathbf{U} >$ is sufficiently regular, it can be (Jordan block) diagonalized using the matrix of its column eigenvectors $\mathbf{Q}$:

$$\mathbf{Q}X_{t+1} = (\mathbf{Q} < \mathbf{U} > \mathbf{Q}^{-1})\mathbf{Q}X_t + \mathbf{Q}\epsilon_{t+1}, \qquad (10.10)$$

or equivalently as

$$Y_{t+1} = < \mathbf{J} > Y_t + W_{t+1}. \qquad (10.11)$$

$Y_t \equiv \mathbf{Q}X_t, W_{t+1} \equiv \mathbf{Q}\epsilon_{t+1}$, and $< \mathbf{J} > \equiv \mathbf{Q} < \mathbf{U} > \mathbf{Q}^{-1}$ is a (block) diagonal matrix in terms of the eigenvalues of $< \mathbf{U} >$.

Thus the (rate distorted) writing of structured stress on the HPA axis through $\delta \mathbf{U}_{t+1}$ is reexpressed in terms of the vector W_{t+1}.

The sequence of W_{t+1} is the rate-distorted image of the information source defined by the system of external structured psychosocial stress. This formulation permits estimation of the long-term steady-state effects of that image on the HPA axis. The basic idea is to recognize that because everything is APSE, we can either time- or ensemble-average both sides of Eq. (10.11), so that the one-period offset is absorbed in the averaging, giving an 'equilibrium' relation

$$< Y >=< \mathbf{J} >< Y > + < W >$$

or

$$< Y >= (\mathbf{I} - < \mathbf{J} >)^{-1} < W >, \qquad (10.12)$$

where $\mathbf{I}$ is the $n \times n$ identity matrix.

Now reverse the argument: suppose that Y_k is chosen to be some fixed eigenvector of $< \mathbf{U} >$. Using the diagonalization of $< \mathbf{J} >$ in terms of its eigenvalues, the average excitation of the HPA axis in terms of some eigentransformed pattern of exciting perturbations becomes

$$< Y_k >= \frac{1}{1- < \lambda_k >} < W_k >, \qquad (10.13)$$

where $< \lambda_k >$ is the eigenvalue of $< Y_k >$, and $< W_k >$ is some appropriately transformed set of ongoing perturbations by structured psychosocial stress.

The essence of this result is that *there will be a characteristic form of perturbation by structured psychosocial stress – the W_k – that will resonantly excite a particular eigenmode of the HPA axis.* Conversely, by tuning the eigenmodes of $< \mathbf{U} >$, the HPA axis can be trained to galvanized response in the presence of particular forms of perturbation.

This is because, if $< \mathbf{U} >$ has been appropriately determined from regression relations, then the λ_k will be a kind of multiple correlation coefficient (Wallace and Wallace, 2000), so that particular eigenpatterns of perturbation will have greatly amplified impact on the behavior of the HPA axis. If $\lambda = 0$ then perturbation has no more effect than its own magnitude.If, however, $\lambda \to 1$, then the written image of a perturbing psychosocial stressor will have very great effect on the HPA axis. Following Ives (1995), call a system with $\lambda \approx 0$ *resilient*, since its response is no greater than the perturbation itself.

10.4   Flight, Fight, and Helplessness

The trained, galvanized, HPA axis response appears to be an evolutionary adaptation to an information theoretic constraint as fundamental as the ubiquity of noise and crosstalk. The argument is fairly intuitive.

Following the direction of Chapter 6 and Sections 3.2–3.4, real-time dynamic responses of an organism involve high probability paths connecting 'initial' multivariate states $\mathbf{S}_0$ to 'final' configurations $\mathbf{S}_f$, across a great variety of beginning and end points. This creates a similar variety of groupoid classifications and associated dual cognitive processes in which the equivalence of two states is defined by linkages to the same beginning and end states. Thus, it becomes possible to construct a 'groupoid free energy' driven by the quality of information coming from the embedding ecosystem, say $\mathcal{H}$, as the temperature analog, extending the pattern of Section 3.4.

This provides an analog to Eq. (6.5): for the dual information source associated with groupoid element G_i, the probability of H_{G_i} becomes

$$P[H_{G_i}] = \frac{\exp[-H_{G_i}/\kappa\mathcal{H}]}{\sum_j \exp[-H_{G_j}/\kappa\mathcal{H}]}, \tag{10.14}$$

defining a free energy Morse function measure as

$$Z_G \equiv -\kappa\mathcal{H}\log[\sum_j \exp[-H_{G_j}/\kappa\mathcal{H}]]. \tag{10.15}$$

This permits a Landau-analog phase transition analysis in which the quality of incoming information from the embedding ecosystem serves to raise or lower the possible richness of an organism's cognitive response to patterns of challenge or opportunity. If $\mathcal{H}$ is relatively large – a rich and varied environment – then there is a plethora of possible cognitive responses. If, however, noise or simple constraint limit the magnitude of $\mathcal{H}$, then the system collapses in a highly punctuated manner to a set of 'ground states' in which only limited responses are possible. Something like an HPA axis, that has been conditioned to respond in a structured but galvanized manner to such limitation, then becomes an important survival tool.

The canonical example, certainly, would be attack from a predator, first under a circumstance where fog-of-war limits accurate perception of threat or detection by the predator, and second, where predation is clearly at hand, but possible responses are few. In each case, $\mathcal{H}$ is quite small, first, limited by noise, and second, by action constraint.

Figure 10.1 shows $\mathcal{H}$ for a two-state system having probabilities $p, q = (1 - p)$ as a function of p. Ground state collapse occurs for $p = 0, 1$, while the richest environment – highest 'temperature' – occurs at $p = 1/2$.

Such 'ground state collapse' must be ubiquitous for real-time cognitive systems facing threat, and can be shown to affect even highly parallel real-time machine cognition. That is, machines that must regulate traffic systems, nuclear reactors, individual vehicle direction, power, communication, and financial grids, and the like, will not have had the relentless benefit of half a billion years of evolutionary selection under circumstances of ground state collapse: their equivalents of the HPA axis are not likely to be particularly well designed.

However, an essential contributor to the human dominance of the planet is our ability to construct cultural systems and artifacts that limit the necessity of even a highly evolved and skilled HPA axis response, as described in the next section.

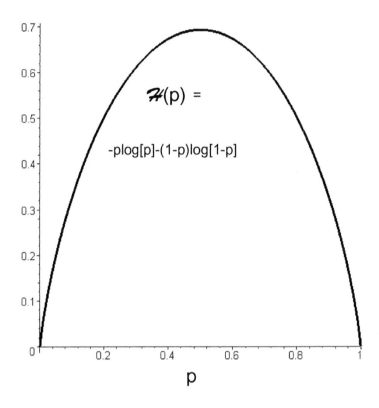

Fig. 10.1   The richness of incoming environmental information for a two-state system, $\mathcal{H} = -p\log[p] - (1-p)\log[1-p]$, as a function of p. The limits of fog-of-war, $p = 0$, and certain attack, $p = 1$, have lowest $\mathcal{H}$, while $p = 1/2$ presents the richest environment. These limits produce two possible 'ground state' condensations.

10.5   Institutions as Niche Construction

Something of the way social structures influence human health can be illustrated by a relatively simple model in which development of a human phenotype adequate to meet environmental demands is 'lubricated' by niche construction provided by embedding institutions.

A multifactorial environmental signal, a 'message', $y^n = \{y_1, y_1, ..., y_n\}$, the systematic output of an embedding ecosystem information source, is expressed by a cognitive genetic or epigenetic expression information source in terms of a multifactorial pattern of organism phenotypes, the 'message' $b^n = \{b_1, b_2, ..., b_n\}$. Assume it possible to deterministically retranslate, 'decode', the phenotype message to produce a new version of the original environmental message, i.e., the environment inferred from the phenotype spectrum. Write that inferred picture as $\hat{y}^n = \{\hat{y}_1, \hat{y}_2\}, ..., \hat{y}_n\}$. Next, introduce a numerical distortion measure that compares y_i with $\hat{y}_i$, writing it as $d(y_i, \hat{y}_i)$. As Cover and Thomas (2006) indicate, many such measures are possible and have been used, and the essential dynamics are, remarkably, independent of the precise measure chosen.

To reiterate, suppose that with each path y^n and b^n-path retranslation into the y language, $\hat{y}^n$, there are associated individual, joint, and conditional probability distributions $p(y^n), p(\hat{y}^n), p(y^n, \hat{y}^n), p(y^n | \hat{p}^n)$.

The average distortion is defined as $D = \sum_{y^n} p(y^n) d(y^n, \hat{y}^n)$.

Clearly, D is an inverse fitness measure: phenotypes that match environments produce higher rates of survival, in this model.

Recall that the rate distortion function, $R(D)$, for a source Y with a distortion measure $d(y, \hat{y})$ is defined as

$$R(D) = \min_{p(y,\hat{y}); \sum_{(y,\hat{y})} p(y)p(y|\hat{y})d(y,\hat{y}) \leq D} I(Y, \hat{Y}).$$

The minimization is over all conditional distributions $p(y|\hat{y})$ for which the joint distribution $p(y, \hat{y}) = p(y)p(y|\hat{y})$ satisfies the average distortion constraint (i.e., average distortion $\leq D$).

The rate distortion theorem states that $R(D)$ is the minimum necessary rate of information transmission that ensures the communication between the interacting entities or systems does not exceed average distortion D. Thus, $R(D)$ defines a minimum necessary channel capacity.

$R(D)$ is, as has been discussed at length, a free energy measure, constrained by the availability of metabolic free energy. As a first approximation, it is possible to write a probability density function for R – a direct fitness measure – as driven by the classic Gibbs relation

$$\exp[-R/Q(\kappa M)], \tag{10.16}$$

where $Q(\kappa M)$ is a monotonic increasing function of available free energy intensity M, with $Q(0) = 0$.

Then

$$P[R] = \frac{\exp[-R/Q(\kappa M)]}{\int_0^\infty \exp[-R/Q(\kappa M)]dR}, \tag{10.17}$$

where κ is an index of the efficiency of use of available metabolic energy rate M.

Higher κM, in this model, permits lower average distortion, and the mean of the average distortion – again, an inverse index of fitness – can be calculated as a function of κM.

For the Gaussian channel, having $R(D) = 1/2 \log[\sigma^2/D]$, so that $D(R) = \sigma^2 \exp[-2R]$, direct calculation gives

$$< D_G >= \int D(R)P[R]dR = \frac{\sigma^2}{2Q(\kappa M) + 1} . \tag{10.18}$$

Note here that if, for example, $Q(\kappa M) = \sqrt[n]{\kappa M}$, then

$$\kappa M = [\frac{1}{2}(\frac{\sigma^2}{< D >} - 1)]^n , \tag{10.19}$$

and high fitness – small $< D >$ – can require enormous rates of metabolic free energy, if σ^2 is not very small.

According to this model, $< D >$, representing an inverse fitness measure, that is, how well a developing organism can represent environmental signals through phenotype expression, depends on both critical internal parameters such as σ^2, and on the exact form of $Q(\kappa M)$.

This result has significant implications for understanding niche construction, that is, using artifacts to decrease σ^2. In the sense of a recent treatment of intrinsically disordered proteins in a rough folding funnel (Wallace, 2011a), niche construction 'self-lubricates' or impedance-matches the relation between genetic and epigenetic expression and environmental demands: decreasing σ^2 reduces the expenditure of metabolic free energy needed to lower D, and hence to increase fitness.

For humans, a central function of social groupings, culture, and larger scale institutions, is to impedance-match phenotype expression to environmental phenotype demand. For Northern cities, those individuals lacking access to winter coats and heated dwellings – the 'homeless' – will suffer markedly diminished lifespans.

10.6   The Hall of Mirrors

Equation (10.6) provides a simple picture of therapeutic intervention as an idiotypic sequence of interventions that brings a pathological dynamic state back toward a normal mode. Intervention causes internal system change that, in turn, alters system output. The potential complexity of this hall of mirrors – the inevitable spectrum of 'side effects' – becomes clearer through an explicit rate distortion calculation.

Recall something of the arguments of Section 6.7. Suppose the relation between system challenge and system response – the manner in which physiological activities of the cognome more-or-less accurately reflect what is called for by environmental conditions – is characterized by a Gaussian channel having a rate distortion function $R(D) = 1/2 \log[\sigma^2/D]$, where D is an average distortion measure based on the squared distortion metric. Defining a rate distortion entropy as the Legendre transform $S_R = R(D) - D dR/dD$ permits definition of a nonequilibrium Onsager equation in the presence of a therapeutic intervention δT as

$$dD/dt = -\mu dS_R/dD - \delta T = \frac{\mu}{2D} - \delta T, \qquad (10.20)$$

having the equilibrium solution, where $dD/dt = 0$,

$$D_{equilib} = \frac{\mu}{2\delta T}. \qquad (10.21)$$

For this simplistic model, the distortion between physiological need and actual physiological response is inversely proportional to the magnitude of therapeutic intervention. In reality, the final distortion measure D is the consequence of a vast array of internal processes that all contribute to it and that, individually, must all be optimized for the organism to survive. That is, overall distortion between total need and total response cannot be constrained by allowing critical subsystems to overload beyond survivable limits: too high a blood pressure spike in response to a stress spike can be fatal.

Consider individual responses of the components of the cognome, for the moment, to be a set of m independent but not identically distributed normal random variates having zero mean and variance $\sigma_i^2, i = 1...m$. Following the argument of Section 10.3.3 of Cover and Thomas (2006), assume a fixed channel capacity R available with which to represent this random vector. How should we allot signal to the various components to minimize the total distortion D? A brief argument shows it necessary to optimize

$$R(D) = \min_{\sum D_i = D} \sum_{i=1}^{m} \max\{1/2 \log[\sigma_i^2/D_i], 0\}, \qquad (10.22)$$

subject to the inequality restraint $\sum_i D_i \leq D$.

Using the Kuhn–Tucker generalization of the Lagrange multiplier method necessary under inequality conditions gives

$$R(D) = \sum_{i=1}^{m} 1/2 \log[\sigma_i^2/D_i], \qquad (10.23)$$

where $D_i = \lambda$ if $\lambda < \sigma_i^2$ or $D = \sigma_i^2$ if $\lambda \geq \sigma_i^2$, and λ is chosen so that $\sum_i D_i = D$.

Thus, even under conditions of 'independence', there is a complex 're-verse water-filling' relation for Gaussian variables. In the real world, the different subcomponents will engage in complicated crosstalk.

Assume m different subsystems that are not independent. Define a rate distortion function $R(D_1, ..., D_m) = R(\mathbf{D})$ and an associated rate distortion entropy S_R having the now-familiar form

$$S_R = R(\mathbf{D}) - \sum_j D_j \partial S_R / \partial D_j \,. \tag{10.24}$$

The generalization of Eq. (10.20) is

$$dD_i/dt = - \sum_j L_{i,j} \partial S_R / \partial D_j - \delta T_i \,. \tag{10.25}$$

At equilibrium, all $dD_i/dt \equiv 0$, so that it becomes necessary to minimize *each* D_i under the joint constraints

$$[\sum_j L_{i,j} \partial S_R / \partial D_j] + \delta T_i = 0 \,,$$

$$D_i \leq D_i^{max} \,\forall i \,, \tag{10.26}$$

remembering that $R(\mathbf{D})$ must be a convex function.

The D_i^{max} represent limits on both internal and external distortion measures as needed for survival.

This is a complicated problem in Kuhn–Tucker optimization for which the exact form of the crosstalk-dominated $R(\mathbf{D})$ is quite unknown, in the context that even the independent Gaussian channel example involves constraints of mutual influence via reverse water-filling. In sum, changing a single therapeutic intervention δT_i will inevitably reverberate across the entire system, necessarily affecting – sometimes markedly – each distortion measure that characterizes the difference between needed and observed physiological subsystem response to challenge.

There may, in fact, be no general solution having $D_i \leq D_i^{max} \forall\, i$.

Side effects are, then, inevitable for therapeutic intervention. Many will be serious. Some will be fatal.

10.7   Side Effects Reconsidered

Sections 10.2 and 10.6 examined adverse reactions to therapeutic intervention – side effects – in a highly formal manner. It is worth explicitly restating the argument from another perspective.

Wallace (2008b, 2009b, 2010b) has examined programming and stability of massively parallel, autonomic 'Self-X' computing systems that will be expected to program, protect, and repair themselves while managing critical duties in real time. Massively parallel real-time systems are inherently coevolutionary, in the sense of the work here, since decisions and choices within one sector inevitably affect the operation of other sectors.

Programming such machines, in the view of those papers, involves 'farming' them via large deviations imposed by the programmer, and allowing the machine itself to concentrate on meeting the goals set by the farmer.

In short, although such machines will soon be deployed to manage many socially important tasks, we do not know how to program or stabilize them: they have not had the benefit of nearly a billion years of evolutionary selection to prune out architectures unsuited to their imposed, ecologically defined, task set. Indeed, the large deviations arguments show that programming and stability for these devices are locked into a duality, an idiotypic and reflective mutuality that implies it is as hard to stabilize as to program them.

Problems facing the medical farming of the human cognome are recognizably similar. While the normal function of that massively parallel system reflects a billion years of mutual fine tuning between embedding ecosystem and the cognome, via selection and interaction pressures, the imposition of institutionally approved medical interventions is quite new, on evolutionary timescales. The inherent duality between programming and stability for massively parallel coevolutionary systems implies that every medical treatment, at any scale, will have 'side effects' that represent the difficulty in stabilizing the system after perturbation. Sections 10.2 and 10.6 suggest some of these difficulties can be examined as a kind of idiotypic 'hall of mirrors'.

To reiterate the discussion in even less formal terms, Lazarou *et al.* (1998) suggest that drug side effects are already the fourth commonest cause of death in the US. In addition, adverse drug reactions, to paraphrase Pirmohamed *et al.* (2002), are typically either consistent with the known pharmacology of the drug, representing an augmentation of its known effects, and are dose-dependent, or else are bizarre responses to idiosyncratic induced hypersensitivity, with highly variable outcomes depending on both the drug and the patient.

The essential role of stress in drug efficacy was recognized some time ago by Downing and Rickels (1982), work rediscovered recently by Haller and colleagues (Haller and Halasz, 2000; Haller, 2001). Downing and Rickels found that the anxiolytic efficacy of chlordiazepoxide and diazepam was markedly reduced in patients experiencing unfavorable life events during drug treatment, compared with both patients experiencing favorable life events or no major events. As Haller (2001) put it:

> To our knowledge, the impact of this finding [i.e., Downing and Rickels, (1982)] was relatively small, and animal research on the topic was not prompted by it... [nonetheless] these and other similar findings show that drug efficacy is not constant, and [epi]genetic factors (e.g., stress) have a strong modulator effect.

Patient medication noncompliance, to paraphrase the conventional perspective taken by Miura *et al.* (2001), is already a serious factor limiting the effectiveness of medical treatments. For instance, the classic study of Sackett and Haynes (1976), found that, even under the best of circumstances, over 30 percent of patients skipped their prescribed doses regardless of their disease, prognosis, or symptoms.

Many such problems are related to maintaining long-term therapy in patients with chronic disease such as hypertension. Factors encouraging noncompliance in long-term therapy include the cost of medication, lack of written instructions, nonparticipation of the patient in designing the treatment plan, lack of patient education about disease, side effects, and inconvenient dosing schedules. These factors may enhance the frequency of patient noncompliance as the duration of drug therapy is prolonged.

Langer (1999) takes a view more in concert with current medical anthropology:

> Care providers [have socially constructed] behavior as compliant when it was patterned by their expectations and noncompliant when behavior deviated from their [culturally and socially conditioned] expectations... [Their] [l]ack of awareness of cultural issues increases [patient-provider] social distance, breaks down communications, and precipitates misconceptions between minority patients and their health care providers. Therefore, opportunities for patient dissatisfaction and noncompliance increase...

> Brock and Salinsky (1993) use the term therapeutic alliance to denote a process in which the health care provider communicates an assessment of the patient's problem and coordinates a practical management plan that is conducive to patient compliance. This assessment must consider and integrate information about all the

systems in which the person exists: biological, psychological, informal/formal social support system, and cultural... Elevating the patient's status within the therapeutic alliance increases the likelihood of...participation, that is, enhanced compliance.

Stress is not undifferentiated, like pressure under water, but often has a complicated grammar and syntax that can, in a sense, carve a distorted image of that structure onto basic human physiological and psychological systems, and on their responses to medical intervention, including but not limited to, pharmaceuticals.

These ideas can be, quite formally, synthesized at and across physiological, psychological, and psychosocial levels of organization, particularly considering the impact of structured stress on the therapeutic alliance.

Essential clues are likely to be found in observed patterns of population-level disparity in drug efficacy, adverse reactions, and compliance across ethnic groups, once contemporary pharmacogenetic ideology has been discounted.

How do structured psychosocial stress and the institutions that moderate or impose it actually affect disease onset and progression and the effectiveness of therapeutic intervention? Two case histories constitute the following chapter.

Chapter 11

HISTORY AND HEALTH

Psychosocial stress can write an image of itself on development at different levels of organization and on different scales of time. Historical patterns of stress, in particular, leave indelible marks on populations that can cause them to respond differently to both medical interventions and to relatively short duration stressors.

Here are two examples that represent the population-level 'fixing' of the human cognome by patterns of psychosocial stress on both long and short timescales.

11.1 Malaria and the Fulani

Modiano *et al.* (1996, 1998, 2001a, b) conducted comparative surveys on three roughly co-resident West African ethnic groups exposed to the same strains of malaria. The Fulani, Mossi, and Rimaibe live in the same conditions of hyperendemic transmission in a Sudan savanna area northeast of Ouagadougou, Burkina Faso. The Mossi and Rimaibe are Sudanese Negroid populations with a long tradition of sedentary farming, while the Fulani are nomadic pastoralists, partly settled and characterized by non-Negroid features of possible Caucasoid origin.

Parasitological, clinical, and immunological investigations showed consistent interethnic differences in *P. Falciparum* infection rates, malaria morbidity, and prevalence and levels of antibodies to various *P. Falciparum* antigens. The data point to a remarkably similar response to malaria in the Mossi and Rimaibe, while the Fulani are clearly less parasitized, less affected by the disease, and more responsive to all antigens tested. No difference in the use of malaria protective measures was demonstrated that could account for these findings. Known genetic factors of resistance to malaria showed markedly *lower* frequencies in the Fulani (Modiano *et al.*, 2001a, b). The differences in the immune response were not explained by the entomological observations, which indicated substantially uniform exposure to infective bites.

In their first study, Modiano *et al.* (1996) concluded that sociocultural factors are not involved in this disparity, and that the available data support the existence of unknown genetic factors, possibly related to humoral immune responses, determining interethnic differences in the susceptibility to malaria.

In spite of later finding the Fulani in their study region have significantly *reduced* frequencies of the classic malaria-resistance genes compared to the other ethnic groups, Modiano *et al.* (2001a, b) again concluded that their evidence supports the existence in the Fulani of unknown genetic factor(s) of resistance to malaria.

This vision of strict genetic causality carries consequences, seriously constraining interpretation of the efficacy of interventions. Modiano *et al.* (1998) report results of an experiment in their Burkina Faso study zone involving the distribution of permethrin-impregnated curtains (PIC) to the three co-resident populations, with markedly different results:

> The PIC were distributed in June 1996 and their impact on malaria infection was evaluated in [the three] groups whose baseline levels of immunity to malaria differed because of their age and ethnic group. Age- and ethnic-dependent efficacy of the PIC was observed. Among Mossi and Rimaibe, the impact (parasite rate reduction after PIC installation with respect to the pre-intervention surveys) was 18.8 % and 18.5 %, respectively. A more than two-fold general impact (42.8 %) was recorded in the Fulani. The impact of the intervention on infection rates appears positively correlated with the levels of anti-malaria immunity...

Modiano *et al.* (1998) conclude from this experiment that the expected complementary role of a hypothetical vaccine is presaged by these results, which also, in their view, emphasize the importance of the genetic background of the population in the evaluation and application of malaria control strategies.

While their results are important for a hypothetical vaccine, much in the spirit of Lewontin (2000), it is possible to differ with the *ad hoc* presumptions of genetic causality, which paper over alternatives involving environment and development consistent with these observations.

A medical anthropologist, Andrew Gordon (2000), has published a detailed study of Fulani cultural identity and illness:

> Cultural identity – who the Fulani think they are – informs thinking on illnesses they suffer. Conversely, illness, so very prevalent in sub-Saharan Africa, provides Fulani with a consistent reminder of their distinctive condition... How they approach being ill also tells Fulani about themselves. The manner in which Fulani think they are sick expresses their sense of difference from other ethnic groups. Schemas of [individual] illness and of collective identity draw deeply from the same well and web of thoughts... As individuals disclose or conceal illness, as they discuss illness and the problem of others, they reflect standards of Fulani life – being strong of character not necessarily of body, being disciplined, rigorously Moslem, and leaders among lessors...to be in step with others and with cultural norms is to have pride in the self and the foundations of Fulani life.

The Fulani carried the Islamic invasion of Africa into the sub-Sahara, enslaving and deculturing a number of ethnic groups, and replacing the native languages with their own. This is much the way African-Americans were enslaved, decultured, and taught English.

As Gordon puts it:

> 'True Fulani' see themselves as distinguished by their aristocratic descent, religious commitments, and personal qualities that clearly differ from lowland cultivators. Those in the lowland are, historically, Fulani subjects who came to act like and speak Fulani, but they are thought to be without the right genealogical descent. The separation between pastoralists and agriculturists repeats itself in settlements across Africa. The terms vary from place to place in Guinea, the terms are Fulbhe for the nobles and the agriculturalist Bhalebhe or Maatyubhee; in Burkina Faso, Fulbhe and the agricultural Rimaybhe; and in Nigeria, the Red Fulani and the agricultural Black Fulani... The schemas for the Fulani body describe the differences between them and others. These are differences that justify pride in being Fulani and not Bhalebhe, Maatyubhe, Rimaybhe, or Black Fulani. In Guinea, the word 'Bhalebhe' means 'the black one'. The term 'Bhalebhe' carries the same meaning as 'Negro' did for Africans brought to North America. It effaces any tribal identity...

The control a Fulani exercises over the body is an essential feature of 'the Fulani way.' Being out of control is shameful and not at all Fulani-like... To act without restraint is to be what is traditionally thought of as Bhalebhe...

Being afflicted with malaria – and handling it well – is a significant proof of ethnicity. How Fulani handle malaria may be telling. What they lack in physical resistance to disease they make up in persistence. Though sickly, Fulani men only reluctantly give into malaria and forgo work. To give into physical discomfort is not *dimo*. When malaria is severe for a man he is likely not to succumb to bed, but instead to sit outside of his home socializing.

The contrasting Occam's Razor hypothesis to genetic determinism, then, is that the observed significant difference in both malarial parasitization and the efficacy of non-pharmaceutical intervention between the historically dominant Fulani and co-resident historically subordinate ethnic groups in the Ouagadougou region of Burkina Faso is largely accounted for by longitudinal and cross-sectional factors of structured psychosocial stress, synergistically intersecting with medical intervention, particularly in view of the *lower* frequencies of classic malaria-resistance genes found in the Fulani.

It is not that the Fulani are not parasitized, or that the 'Fulani way' prevents disease, but that the population-level burdens of environment are modulated by historical development, and these are profoundly different for former masters and former slaves.

11.2   The American Catastrophe

Both diabetes and hypertension are associated with increased risk for Alzheimer's disease (e.g., Sims-Robinson *et al.*, 2010; Kivipelto *et al.*, 2001), and the 'obesity epidemic' in the US is related to rising rates of both disorders. It is of interest to parse those increases according to White and African-American ethnicity, in accordance with the discussions above.

Two powerful and intertwining phenomena of socioeconomic disintegration – deurbanization in the 1970s, and deindustrialization, particularly since 1980 – have combined to profoundly damage many US communities, dispersing historic accumulations of economic, political, and social capital. These losses have had manifold and persisting impacts on both institutions and individuals (Pappas, 1989; Ullmann, 1988; Wallace and Wallace, 1998).

Wallace *et al.* (1999) examined the effect of these policy-driven phenomena on the hierarchical diffusion of AIDS in the US. That work can be extended to their association with obesity, in the context of Section 6.7.

By 1980, not a single African-American urban community established before or during World War II remained intact. Many Hispanic urban neighborhoods established after the war suffered similar fates. Virtually all lost considerable housing, population, and economic and social capital either to programs of urban renewal in the 1950s or to policy-related contagious urban decay from the late 1960s through the late 1970s (Wallace and Wallace, 2007; Wallace and Wallace, 1998; Wallace and Fullilove, 2008; Fullilove and Wallace, 2011).

Figure 11.1 gives an example, showing the percent change of occupied housing units in the Bronx section of New York City between 1970 and 1980 by Health Area, the aggregation of US Census Tracts by which morbidity and mortality are reported in the city. The South-Central section of the Bronx, by itself one of the largest urban concentrations in the Western world with about 1.4 million inhabitants, lost between 55 and 80% of housing units, most within a five-year period. This is a level of damage unprecedented in an industrialized nation short of civil or international war, and indeed can be construed as a kind of covert civil war aimed at ethnic minority voting blocks (Wallace and Wallace, 1998; Wallace and Fullilove, 2008; Fullilove and Wallace, 2011).

Figure 11.2, a composite index of number and seriousness of building fires from 1959 through 1990 (Wallace and Wallace, 1998; Wallace *et al.*, 1999), illustrates the process of contagious urban decay in New York City producing that housing loss, affecting large sections of Harlem in Manhattan, and a broad band across the African-American and Hispanic neighborhoods of Northern Brooklyn, from Williamsburg to Bushwick, Brownsville, and East New York. The sudden rise between 1967 and 1968 was stemmed through 1972 by the opening of 20 new fire companies in high fire incidence, minority neighborhoods of the city. Beginning in late 1972, however, some 50 firefighting units were closed and many others destaffed as part of a 'planned shrinkage' program that continued the ethnic cleansing policies of 1950s urban renewal without benefit of either constitutional niceties or new housing construction to shelter the displaced population (Wallace and Wallace, 1998; Wallace and Fullilove, 2008; Fullilove and Wallace, 2011).

Similar maps and graphs could be drawn for devastated sections of Detroit, Chicago, Los Angeles, Philadelphia, Baltimore, Cleveland, Pittsburgh, Newark, and a plethora of smaller US urban centers, each with its

PERCENT CHANGE IN OCCUPIED HOUSING 1970-1980

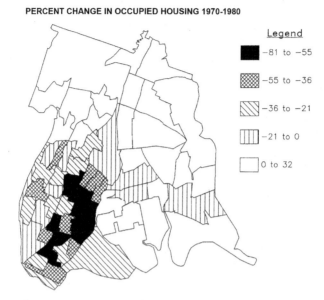

Legend

■ −81 to −55

▦ −55 to −36

▧ −36 to −21

▥ −21 to 0

☐ 0 to 32

Fig. 11.1   Percent change in occupied housing units, Bronx section of New York City, 1970–1980. Large areas lost over half their housing in this period, a degree of destruction unprecedented in an industrialized nation outside of wartime. Similar policy-driven disasters have afflicted most US urban minority communities since the end of World War II.

own individual story of active public policy and passive 'benign neglect'.

Figure 11.1 represents the Bronx part of the spatial distribution of the time integral of Fig. 11.2.

Figure 11.3, using data taken from the US Census, shows the counties of the Northeastern US losing more than 1,000 manufacturing jobs between 1972 and 1987, the famous rust belt. It is, in its way, an exact parallel to Fig. 11.1 in that unionized manufacturing jobs lost remained lost, and their associated social capital and political influence were dispersed. As Pappas (1989) describes, the effects were profound and permanent:

By 1982 mass unemployment had reemerged as a major social issue [in the USA]. Unemployment rose to its highest level since before World War II, and an estimated 12 million people were out of work – 10.8% of the labor force in the nation. It was not, however, a really new phenomenon. After 1968 a pattern was established in which each recession was followed by higher levels of unemployment

NEW YORK CITY FIRE EPIDEMIC
1959-1990

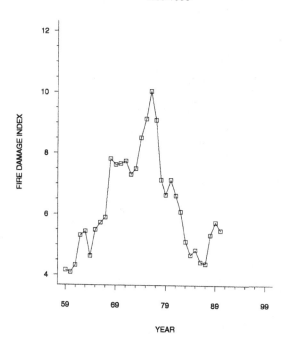

Fig. 11.2   Annual fire damage index, New York City, 1959–1990, a composite of number and seriousness of structural fires, and an index of contagious urban decay. Some 20 new fire companies were added to high fire areas between 1969 and 1971, interrupting the process. Fifty firefighting units were closed in or permanently relocated from, high fire areas after November, 1972, allowing contagious urban decay to proceed to completion, producing the conditions of Fig. 11.1.

during recovery. During the depth of the 1975 recession, national unemployment rose to 9.2%. In 1983, when a recovery was proclaimed, unemployment remained at 9.5% annually.

Certain sectors of the work force have been more heavily affected than others. There was a 16.9% jobless rate among blue-collar workers in April, 1982... Unemployment and underemployment have become major problems for the working class. While monthly unemployment figures rise and fall, these underlying problems have persisted over a long period. Mild recoveries merely distract out attention from them.

Counties Losing More Than 1000 Manufacturing Jobs 1972-87 ☐ COUNTY

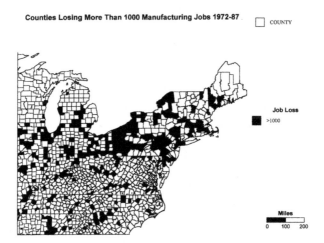

Fig. 11.3   The Rust Belt: counties of the Northeastern US which lost 1,000 or more manufacturing jobs between 1972 and 1987.

Figure 11.4, illustrating data from the US Bureau of Labor Statistics, shows the total number of US manufacturing jobs from 1980 to 2001. We define an environmental index of the US national pattern of structured stress by *the integral of manufacturing job loss after 1980*, i.e., the space between the observed curve and a horizontal line drawn out from the 1980 number of jobs. This is not quite the same as Fig. 11.3, that represents a simple net loss between two time periods. It appears that manufacturing job loss at one period continues to have influence at subsequent periods as a consequence of permanently dispersed social and political capital, at least over a 20-year span.

Other models, perhaps with different integral weighting functions, are possible. The simplest, used here, is

$$\mathcal{D}(T) = -\sum_{\tau=1980}^{\tau=T} \left[M(\tau) - M(1980)\right]. \tag{11.1}$$

A more elaborate treatment might be

$$\mathcal{D}(T) = -\int_{\tau_0}^{T} f(T-\tau)M(\tau)d\tau, \tag{11.2}$$

where $\mathcal{D}$ is the deficit, $M(\tau)$ is the number of manufacturing jobs at time τ, and $f(T-\tau)$ is a lagged weighting function.

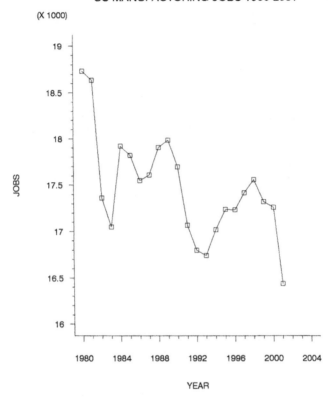

Fig. 11.4   Annual number of manufacturing jobs in the US, 1980–2001. The environmental index of social decay is the integrated loss after the 1980 peak, representing the
permanent dispersal of economic, social, and political capital, part of the opportunity
cost of a deindustrialization largely driven by the diversion of technical resources from
civilian industry into the Cold War (e.g., Ullmann, 1988).

Figure 11.5, using data from the Centers for Disease Control (2003),
shows the percent of US adults characterized as obese according to the
Behavioral Risk Factor Surveillance System between 1991 and 2001. This
is given as a function of the integrated manufacturing jobs deficit from 1980,
again, calculated as a simple negative sum of annual differences from 1980.

The association is quite good indeed, and the theory of Sections 10.3
and 10.4 suggests the relation is causal and not simply correlational: loss of
stable working class employment, loss of social and political capital, loss of
union influence on working conditions and public policies, deurbanization

PERCENT OBESE VS. CUMULATIVE
MANUFACTURING JOBS DEFICIT FROM 1980

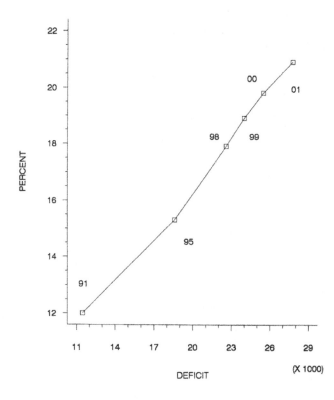

Fig. 11.5   1991–2001 relation between adult obesity in the US and the integrated loss of manufacturing jobs after 1980. Manufacturing job loss is an index of permanent decline in social, economic, and political capital that is perceived as, and indeed represents, a serious threat to the well-being of the US population.

intertwined with deindustrialization and their political outfalls, all constitute a massive threat expressing itself in population-level patterns of HPA axis-driven metabolism and metabolic syndrome. See Bjorntorp (2001) for a more comprehensive exploration of the relation between psychosocial stress and obesity.

Figure 11.6 extends the analysis to diabetes deaths in the US between 1980 and 1998. It shows the death rate per 100,000 as a function of the cumulative manufacturing jobs deficit from 1980 through 1998. Diabetes deaths are, after a lag, a good index of population obesity. Two systems are

evident, before and after 1989, with a phase transition between them probably representing, in Holling's (1973) sense, a change in ecological domain
roughly analogous to the sudden eutrophication of a lake progressively subjected to contaminated runoff. This would seem to reflect the delayed cumulative impacts of both deindustrialization and the deurbanization which
became closely coupled with it. Further sudden, marked, upward transitions seem likely if socioeconomic and political reforms are not forthcoming.
A simple linear correlation for the period gives an R^2 of 0.91.

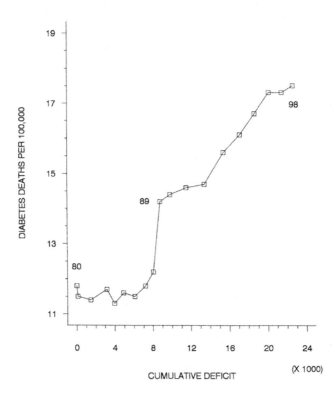

Fig. 11.6   1980–1998 relation between US diabetes death rate and integrated loss of
manufacturing jobs after 1980. Two systems are evident: before and after 1989. We
believe this sudden change represents a nonlinear transition between ecosystem domains
which is much like the eutrophication of an increasingly contaminated water body (e.g.,
Holling, 1973). The simple correlation has $R^2 = 0.91$.

It would be useful to compare annual county-level maps of diabetes, hypertension, Alzheimer's, and Parkinson's disease death rates with those of manufacturing job loss and deurbanization, but such a study would require considerable resources in order to conduct the necessary sophisticated analyses of cross-coupled, lagged, spatial and social diffusion.

Figure 11.7 shows a regression of the Black vs. White diabetes death rates (per 100,000) in the US for the period 1979–1997. It is striking that, while the rate of increase for African-Americans was more than 50% higher than for whites, both subpopulations were closely linked together in a relentless progression: the R^2 of the regression was 0.99. Similarly, Fig. 11.8 shows Black vs. White hypertension death rates (per 100,000) over the same time span. Again, while African-Americans suffered proportionally more than Whites, the two groups were closely linked in a remarkable joint increase, $R^2 = 0.85$.

Diabetes and hypertension are closely related to obesity, and to the onset of Alzheimer's disease. The increased slopes of the regression lines of Figs. 11.7 and 11.8 indicate that death rates of hypertension and diabetes in African-American populations are, respectively, 26 to 53% higher than for Whites over the period 1979-1997, while both increase relentlessly during that period. This pattern suggests that rates of Alzheimer's disease in African-Americans will be similarly, and necessarily, elevated (Alzheimer's Association, 2006).

A pilot study: Alzheimer's disease

Two obvious national indices of the catastrophe implied by Figs. 11.3 and 11.4 are percent unemployed and the percent of the workforce in a union, and it is possible to construct an elementary model of state-level Alzheimer's disease deaths based on them. The dependent variate is the 'young elderly' annual average Alzheimer's death rate (ICD-10 G30 classification) per 100,000 for the age range 65–74 in the period 1999–2006. Data are taken from the CDC Wonder web site. The independent variates are the percent unemployed in 2003, and percent of the workforce union members, 2004, available from the US Department of Labor Statistics.

The 50-state regression model, having F=7.98, P=0.0010, adjusted R^2=22.2%, is given by:

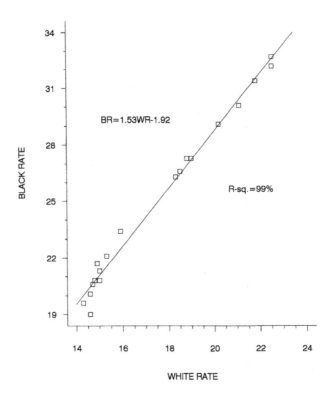

Fig. 11.7   US Black vs. White diabetes death rates (per 10^5), 1979–97. While the Black rates are uniformly higher, strong coupling implies both populations are closely linked in a deteriorating social structure.

Parameter	Estimate	SE	t	P
CONSTANT	18.76	3.86	4.86	0.0000
unemp03	1.407	0.694	2.03	0.048
unionpc04	-0.503	0.132	-3.82	0.0004

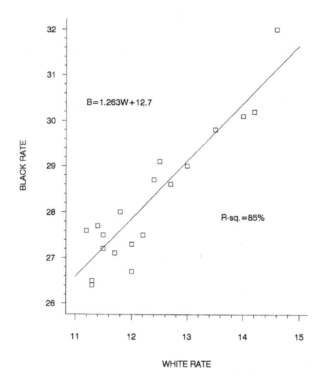

Fig. 11.8   Same as Fig. 11.7 for US hypertension death rates.

The model works, and in the expected direction: union participation indexes a decrease, and unemployment an increase, of Alzheimer's mortality incidence in the young elderly, consistent with a theoretical model for which locus-of-control affects HPA axis activity and the de facto rate of aging, long recognized as the principal 'risk factor' for Alzheimer's disease.

It is, however, possible to parse these results even further: the Southern US states form the core of the so-called 'right-to-work' (RTW) laws that forbid requiring a worker to join a union even if he or she is employed in a work force that has union representation (see Fig. 11.9). RTW laws indicate and instantiate a culture of individualism and of active anti-collectivism. Other differences between the RTW and non-RTW states include economic history with the former relatively recently industrialized and historically agricultural. Indeed, the plains and Southwestern RTW states showed the fastest rate of increase in manufacturing jobs in the 1990s, but very low numbers of such jobs per unit population. Typically, indicators of social and political engagement such as voting participation and percent employed belonging to a union showed large differences between the two groups of states. Together, they likely indicate the strength of social and political support and control within the two groups of states.

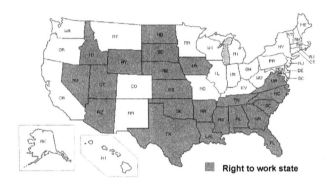

Fig. 11.9 'Right-to-work' states in the USA. These states forbid requiring a worker to join a union even if employed by a workforce that has union representation.

The first step is to examine annual average rates of Alzheimer's deaths per 100,000 over the years 1999–2006 for three age cohorts: 65–74, 75–84, and 85+ across the two sets of states, and compare them using a standard t-test:

Cohort	1	2	3
RTW	23.0	182.2	843.1
Non-RTW	19.3	159.3	802.7
P(t-test)	0.02	0.04	NS

The rates, as expected, increase sharply with cohort age, but are markedly lower at all ages in the non-RTW states, and statistically significantly so in the younger.

The regression model above can be applied to all three cohorts and for the US, RTW, and non-RTW states. The percent of adjusted variance accounted for by the models, R^2, and the maximum significance P of the regressions, is as follows:

Cohort	1	2	3	Max. P
US	22.1	33.0	8.7	0.04
Non-RTW	16.6	31.8	20.8	0.04
RTW	0	12.4	0	NS

Although the RTW regressions are not significant, the others are highly so, and the raw numbers all show a peak in the middle cohort.

Figure 11.10 displays these results as a signal-to-noise ratio vs. signal amplitude graph. Age is taken as a de facto toxic exposure, and the regression adjusted R^2 as the SN measure for the model.

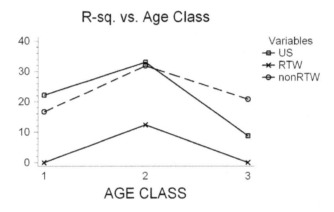

Fig. 11.10   Regression adjusted R^2 as signal-to-noise ratio vs. age cohort as toxic exposure for a model based on percent unemployed and percent of workforce unionized. The SNR follows a unimodal 'inverted U' pattern consistent with signal transduction, with the non-RTW states shifted to higher ages. This is consistent with a biosemiotics perspective in which the degree of physiological meaning of the population-level response to the driving variates is changed by the underlying cultural milieu.

Two essential points are the failure of the model for the RTW states and the relative shift of the non-RTW toward the older cohort relative to the full US model. The inference is that collective efficacy appears to lower an HPA axis-induced premature aging that expresses itself in Alzheimer's mortality in the young elderly, in accordance with theory. Underlying cultural context appears to profoundly affect both the rate of 'effective aging' and the population response to patterns of affordance and stress.

Further work in this direction should be done using data at the county level of analysis – encompassing some 3,800 distinct geographic entities –

to increase the analytic power, illuminate mechanisms at different scales, and explore how policy affects linkages across scales.

A possible inference of these results, partial as they may be, is that Stern's (2009) idea of cognitive reserve may extend to the embedding of the individual in community. That is, in the sense of Wallace and Fullilove (2008), the 'natural' human state includes a powerful measure of distributed cognition that can, in a likely synergistic manner, buffer both cognitive decline and the rate of physiological aging. One implication would be that the RTW states in particular, and the US in general, following the arguments of Heine (2001) and Henrich et al. (2010), embody a pathologically individualistic culture that is contrary to evolved human norms, a disjunction expressing itself in premature aging.

Anti-public health

Current theory clearly identifies stress as critical to the etiology of visceral obesity, the metabolic syndrome, and their pathological sequelae – including protein folding disorders such as Alzheimer's disease – mediated by the HPA axis and other physiological subsystems (Qui et al., 2009; Bjorntorp, 2001).

Both animal and human studies, however, have indicated that not all stressors are equal in their effect: particular forms of domination in animals and lack of control over work activities in humans are well known to be especially effective in triggering metabolic syndrome and chronic inflammatory coronary lipid deposition. Thus stress can be given meaning from context.

Recent analyses have examined the general association between social status and health in Western subcultures. For example, Fig. 11.11, from Singh-Manoux et al. (2003), displays a clear dose-response relation between age adjusted prevalence of self-reported ill-health versus self-reported status rank for white collar workers in the UK. 1 is high rank and 10 is low rank. The low status group approaches the 'LD-50' level at which half the population shows a response to dosage.

For the US, Fig. 11.12 shows the percent of income concentrated in the top 5% of the population as a function of the integral of manufacturing job loss, 1980–1998. The correlation is very high indeed, suggesting that the destruction of the US industrial base consequent on the catastrophic diversion of scientific and engineering resources into the Cold War (e.g., Ullmann, 1988; Wallace, et al., 1999) has had the effect of concentrating wealth and power in the hands of a very small segment of the population. The loss of unionized industrial jobs, and their guarantees of job security, health insurance, retirement benefits, and the exercise of collective power

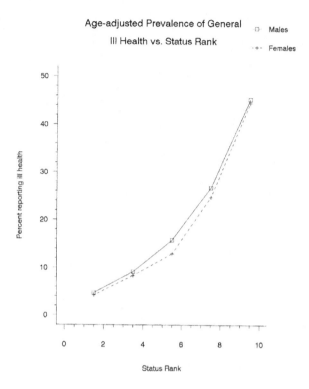

Fig. 11.11 Redisplay of data from Singh-Manoux *et al.* (2003). Sex-specific dose-response curves of age-adjusted self-reported ill-health vs. self-reported status rank, Whitehall II cohort, 1997 and 1999. 1 is high status, 10 is low status. The curve is approaching the LD-50 at which half the dosed population suffers physiological effect of a poison.

seems a principal source of a widening population-level stress that has been concentrated in African-American populations via the familiar pattern of 'last hired, first fired'.

Figure 11.13 shows the simple linear correlation between the annual percent of the US voting age population convicted of a felony between 1980 and 1998 and the integral of manufacturing job loss for the period. The correlation is very good indeed. The percent of felons tripled, serving as yet another index of, and significant contributor to, population level stress.

The analysis has been in terms of a cognitive HPA axis responding in a culturally specific manner to a highly structured 'language' of psychosocial stress. Stress, then, literally writes a distorted image of itself onto the

% OF US INCOME IN TOP 5 % VS INTEGRAL
OF MANUFACTURING JOB LOSS, 1980-98

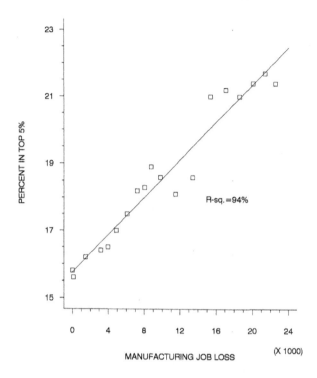

Fig. 11.12   Percent of total US income concentrated in the highest 5% as a function of the integral of manufacturing job loss, 1980–1998. Devastation of the manufacturing sector consequent on the disruptions caused by the Cold War diversion of engineering and scientific resources from the civilian economy has disempowered vast sections of the US population.

behavior of the HPA axis in a way analogous to learning plateaus in a neural network or to punctuated equilibrium in a simple evolutionary process. The first form of phase transition/generalized symmetry change might be regarded as representing the progression of a normally 'staged' disease. The other could describe certain pathologies characterized by stasis or only slight change, with staging a rare (and perhaps fatal) event. The works of Barker and his group (e.g., Barker, 2002; Barker *et al.*, 2002) suggest that

FELONS AS % OF VOTING-AGE POPULATION VS.
INTEGRAL OF MANUFACTURING JOB LOSS 80-98

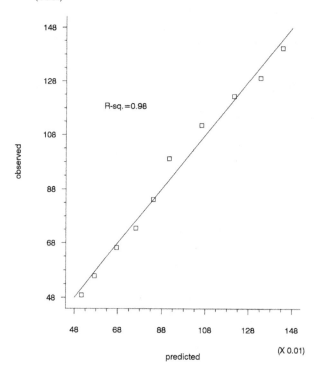

Fig. 11.13 Felons as a percent of the US voting-age population, 1980–1998, expressed as a linear function of the integral of the manufacturing job loss over the period. The proportion of felons tripled. The high correlation suggests that the loss of stable, union-ized, manufacturing jobs in the US affects public order as well as public health, and these deteriorations, of course, are likely to be powerfully synergistic.

such HPA axis dysfunction in a mother can become a strong epigenetic catalyst for her children.

To reiterate, psychosocial stress is, for humans, a culturally specific artifact, one of many such that interact intimately with human physiology. Indeed, much current theory in evolutionary anthropology focuses on the essential (but not unique) role culture plays in human biology (Avital and Jablonka, 2000; Durham, 1991).

If, as the evolutionary anthropologist Robert Boyd has suggested, "Culture is as much a part of human biology as the enamel on our teeth", what does the rising tide of obesity in the US imply about American culture and the American system? About 22% of both African-American and Hispanic children are overweight, as compared to about 12% of non-Hispanic whites, and that prevalence is rising across the board (Strauss and Pollack, 2001). This suggests that, while the effects of an accelerating social pathology related to deindustrialization, deurbanization, and loss of democracy may be most severe for ethnic minorities in the US, the larger, embedding, cultural dysfunction has already spread upward along the social hierarchy, and is quickly entraining the majority population as well. This will, according to analysis, become expressed in rising rates of protein folding and related disorders for majority and minority populations, although not at the same rates.

This explanation, and its policy implications, stand in stark contrast to current individual-oriented exhortations about 'taking responsibility for one's behavior' or 'eating less and getting more exercise' (Hill et al., 2003). Rather, this work implies the fundamental cause of the US obesity epidemic is not television, the automobile, or junk food. All were significant features of American life from the late 1950s into the 1980s without an obesity epidemic. The fundamental cause of the US obesity epidemic is a massive threat to the population caused by continuing deterioration of basic US social and economic structure, including a ratcheting of dominance relations resulting from the concentration of effective power within a shrinking elite. These phenomena are literally writing a life-threatening image of themselves onto the bodies of Americans of all ages through a vast array of illnesses related to the metabolic syndrome (Bjorntorp, 2001). There is a large and growing literature on other aspects of the sharpening inequalities within the US system (particularly Wilkinson, 1996, and related material), and our conclusions fit within that body of work.

The fundamental and highly plastic nature of the biological relation between structured psychosocial stress and the nested set of cognitive physiological systems – the human cognome – ensures that scale-limited magic bullet interventions will be largely circumvented. In the presence of a continuing socioeconomic and political ratchet, simplistic magic bullet medical modalities can provide little more than the equivalent of a choice of death by hanging or firing squad: stress wins however it needs to.

Effective intervention against disorders of the human cognome is predicated on creation of a broad, multilevel, ecological control program – in effect, a large, mulitscale, multilevel, policy-driven 'magic strategy' that transcends magic bullet thinking. It is evident that such a program must include redress of the power relations between groups, rebuilding of urban (and, increasingly, suburban) minority communities, and effective reindustrialization. This implies the necessity of a resurgence of the labor union, religious, civil rights, and community-based political activities which have been traditionally directed against cultural patterns of injustice in the past, activities which, ultimately, liberate all.

In the sense of Heine (2001) and Wallace and Fullilove (2008), the focus in this section has been on the larger historical and cultural contexts of human cognome disorders. These contexts include epigenetic and life-history stress factors related to large-scale public policies that can act as catalysts to induce highly structured 'large deviations' that accelerate the deterioration of the human cognome from the individual to the population level. And we have done this from the ground up, as it were, providing a 'basic biological' model of what Qui *et al.* (2009) and others have observed. The work provides a powerful argument that narrow focus on medical magic bullets is not consonant with the wide scale of physiological and psychosocial dysfunction in the US, and a successful search for effective interventions will necessarily involve far broader perspectives than seem comfortable to the strongly culture-bound majority of senior American researchers and the policymaking elites that employ them.

Chapter 12

BEYOND GLASPERLENSPIEL

A broad spectrum of versions of Bernard Baars' global broadcast model applies to many interacting 'low level' cognitive biological submodules, usually having much longer characteristic time constants than the 100 ms of consciousness for which the construct was initially intended. Generalized global broadcasts, via the giant component linking 'unconscious' cognitive modules, emerge directly via crosstalk linkages, and the effects of external signals and internal 'biological ruminations' can be incorporated through standard arguments leading to punctuated threshold detection.

Thus, the spandrel of inevitable crosstalk between low level cognitive modules becomes a sufficient condition for evolutionary exaptation into the arch of global broadcasts through the information theory chain rule that implies it takes more metabolic free energy to prevent signal correlation than to allow it. Such generalization of neural consciousness, in terms of tunable, shifting global broadcasts, seems ubiquitous, as collective phenomena like wound healing, gene expression, and similar processes imply (Wallace and Wallace, 2010).

Thus, not only is the living state characterized by cognition at every scale and level of organization, but also by multiple, shifting, tunable, cooperative broadcasts analogous to, if more general than, animal consciousness, at and across those same structures (Wallace, 2012c).

This perspective on the human cognome, of an inherently multiscale and multilevel, interactive, and highly dynamic system, has profound implications for Western medicine. From the viewpoint of this study, the solution to the conundrum of Fig. 1.1 is not 'translational medicine' – i.e., more of the same but better. Rather, what is required is a profound reconfiguration of interventions so as to encapsulate more than a single scale or level of organization. That is, it has now become necessary to expand fundamental, underlying perspectives in medicine, moving beyond reductionist small molecule design and overfocus on cellular process, to the principled construction of more comprehensive multifactorial or multiscale interventions. These would be designed to affect the interaction of complementary information source networks, driving them from pathological to benign conformations. The tool would be a 'farming' by externally-imposed, cleverly constructed 'large deviations' in the sense of Eq. (3.5), as expanded in the section on therapeutic intervention. In sum, biomedical research and the design of interventions must shift primary focus from the molecular and cellular to higher levels of organization that include sociocultural context.

At the individual scale, this would appear to require seeking synergistic total treatments, rather than simply applying magic bullets in a traditionally decontextualizing strategy that often attempts to explicitly ignore the embedding social, cultural, and historical processes that sculpt the human cognome.

At the population scale, where public policy can be most effective, the increasing expense of individual level interventions – even if the rate of decline of Fig. 1.1 can be mitigated by following a multiscale or multilevel perspective at the individual level – would seem to imply the necessity of again recognizing what has been known for the last two hundred years, that patterns of health and illness are determined by living and working conditions and the power relations between groups (e.g., Kleinman, Das and Lock, 1994; Wallace and Fullilove, 2008; Wallace and Wallace, 2010).

This is, of course, a difficult tectonic shift in perspective, research strategy, and practice that is likely to be particularly resisted by those trapped at the top of pathological power relations between individuals and groups.

In a sense, Fig. 1.1 represents a bottleneck similar to that facing the computer industry's attempts to increase single-core microprocessor clock rates beyond 3 GHz. Heating from energy dissipation is forcing the manufacture and deployment of massively parallel multicore CPUs. The central bottleneck then becomes the difficult synergistic relation between the programming and stabilizing of such parallel systems (Borkar, 2007; Patterson, 2010). For the inherently massively parallel human cognome, this difficulty is significantly mitigated by a human hypersociality (Richerson and Boyd, 2006) that dictates a small world network in which sociocultural and institutional factors greatly dominate, simplifying, in concept, the design of therapeutic strategies (Fanon, 1966; Memmi, 1967, 1969).

Absent a fundamental shift, from individual treatment to multiscale intervention that recognizes the dominance of psychosocial, cultural, socioeconomic, and institutional structures and trajectories in human health and illness, Western medicine's exponential cost catastrophe will become the wall against which the reductionist biomedical *Glasperlenspiel* will shatter.

Chapter 13

MATHEMATICAL APPENDIX

13.1 The Tuning Theorem

Messages from an information source, seen as symbols x_j from some alphabet, each having probabilities P_j associated with a random variable X, are 'encoded' into the language of a 'transmission channel', a random variable Y with symbols y_k, having probabilities P_k, possibly with error. Someone receiving the symbol y_k then retranslates it (without error) into some x_k, which may or may not be the same as the x_j that was sent.

More formally, the message sent along the channel is characterized by a random variable X having the distribution

$$P(X = x_j) = P_j, j = 1, ..., M.$$

The channel through which the message is sent is characterized by a second random variable Y having the distribution

$$P(Y = y_k) = P_k, k = 1, ..., L.$$

Let the joint probability distribution of X and Y be defined as

$$P(X = x_j, Y = y_k) = P(x_j, y_k) = P_{j,k}$$

and the conditional probability of Y given X as

$$P(Y = y_k | X = x_j) = P(y_k | x_j).$$

Then, the Shannon uncertainty of X and Y independently and the joint uncertainty of X and Y together are defined respectively as

$$H(X) = -\sum_{j=1}^{M} P_j \log(P_j)$$

$$H(Y) = -\sum_{k=1}^{L} P_k \log(P_k)$$

$$H(X,Y) = -\sum_{j=1}^{M}\sum_{k=1}^{L} P_{j,k} \log(P_{j,k}) . \tag{13.1}$$

The *conditional uncertainty* of Y given X is defined as

$$H(Y|X) = -\sum_{j=1}^{M}\sum_{k=1}^{L} P_{j,k} \log[P(y_k|x_j)] . \tag{13.2}$$

For any two stochastic variates X and Y, $H(Y) \geq H(Y|X)$, as knowledge of X generally gives some knowledge of Y. Equality occurs only in the case of stochastic independence.

Since $P(x_j, y_k) = P(x_j)P(y_k|x_j)$, then $H(X|Y) = H(X,Y) - H(Y)$.

The information transmitted by translating the variable X into the channel transmission variable Y – possibly with error – and then retranslating without error the transmitted Y back into X is defined as

$$I(X|Y) \equiv H(X) - H(X|Y) = H(X) + H(Y) - H(X,Y) . \tag{13.3}$$

Again, see Ash (1990), Cover and Thomas (2006), or Khinchin (1957) for details. The essential point is that if there is no uncertainty in X given the channel Y, then there is no loss of information through transmission. In general, this will not be true, and herein lies the essence of the theory.

Given a fixed vocabulary for the transmitted variable X, and a fixed vocabulary and probability distribution for the channel Y, we may vary the probability distribution of X in such a way as to maximize the information sent. The capacity of the channel is defined as

$$C \equiv \max_{P(X)} I(X|Y) , \tag{13.4}$$

subject to the subsidiary condition that $\sum P(X) = 1$.

The critical trick of the Shannon coding theorem for sending a message with arbitrarily small error along the channel Y at any rate $R < C$ is to encode it in longer and longer 'typical' sequences of the variable X; that is, those sequences whose distribution of symbols approximates the probability distribution $P(X)$ above which maximizes C.

If $S(n)$ is the number of such 'typical' sequences of length n, then

$$\log[S(n)] \approx nH(X),$$

where $H(X)$ is the uncertainty of the stochastic variable defined above. Some consideration shows that $S(n)$ is much less than the total number of possible messages of length n. Thus, as $n \to \infty$, only a vanishingly small fraction of all possible messages is meaningful in this sense. This observation, after some considerable development, is what allows the coding theorem to work so well. In sum, the prescription is to encode messages in typical sequences, which are sent at very nearly the capacity of the channel. As the encoded messages become longer and longer, their maximum possible rate of transmission without error approaches channel capacity as a limit. Again, the standard references provide details.

This approach can be, in a sense, inverted to give a tuning theorem variant of the coding theorem.

Telephone lines, optical wave guides, and the tenuous plasma through which a planetary probe transmits data to earth may all be viewed in traditional information-theoretic terms as a *noisy channel* around which we must structure a message so as to attain an optimal error-free transmission rate.

Telephone lines, wave guides, and interplanetary plasmas are, relatively speaking, fixed on the timescale of most messages, as are most sociogeographic networks. Indeed, the capacity of a channel is defined by varying the probability distribution of the 'message' process X so as to maximize $I(X|Y)$.

Suppose there is some message X so critical that its probability distribution must remain fixed. The trick is to fix the distribution $P(x)$ but *modify the channel* – i.e., tune it – so as to maximize $I(X|Y)$. The *dual* channel capacity C^* can be defined as

$$C^* \equiv \max_{P(Y),P(Y|X)} I(X|Y). \tag{13.5}$$

But

$$C^* = \max_{P(Y),P(Y|X)} I(Y|X),$$

since

$$I(X|Y) = H(X) + H(Y) - H(X,Y) = I(Y|X).$$

Thus, in a purely formal mathematical sense, *the message transmits the channel*, and there will indeed be, according to the coding theorem, a channel distribution $P(Y)$ which maximizes C^*.

One may do better than this, however, by modifying the channel matrix $P(Y|X)$. Since

$$P(y_j) = \sum_{i=1}^{M} P(x_i)P(y_j|x_i),$$

$P(Y)$ is entirely defined by the channel matrix $P(Y|X)$ for fixed $P(X)$ and

$$C^* = \max_{P(Y),P(Y|X)} I(Y|X) = \max_{P(Y|X)} I(Y|X).$$

Calculating C^* requires maximizing the complicated expression

$$I(X|Y) = H(X) + H(Y) - H(X,Y),$$

which contains products of terms and their logs, subject to constraints that the sums of probabilities are 1 and each probability is itself between 0 and 1. Maximization is done by varying the channel matrix terms $P(y_j|x_i)$ within the constraints. This is a difficult problem in nonlinear optimization. However, for the special case $M = L$, C^* may be found by inspection. If $M = L$, then choose

$$P(y_j|x_i) = \delta_{j,i}$$

where $\delta_{i,j}$ is 1 if $i = j$ and 0 otherwise. For this special case

$$C^* \equiv H(X)$$

with $P(y_k) = P(x_k)$ for all k. Information is thus transmitted without error when the channel becomes 'typical' with respect to the fixed message distribution $P(X)$.

If $M < L$ matters reduce to this case, but for $L < M$ information must be lost, leading to rate distortion limitations.

Thus modifying the channel may be a far more efficient means of ensuring transmission of an important message than encoding that message in a 'natural' language which maximizes the rate of transmission of information on a fixed channel.

We have examined the two limits in which either the distributions of $P(Y)$ or of $P(X)$ are kept fixed. The first provides the usual Shannon coding theorem, and the second a tuning theorem variant, i.e., a tunable, retina-like, rate distortion manifold, in the sense of Glazebrook and Wallace (2009a, b).

Indeed, this result is well known using another description. Following Chiang and Boyd (2004), Shannon (1959) wrote:

There is a curious and provocative duality between the properties of [an information] source with a distortion measure and those of a channel. This duality is enhanced if we consider channels in which there is a cost associated with the different letters... Solving this problem corresponds, in a sense, to finding a source that is right for the channel and the desired cost... In a somewhat dual way, evaluating the rate distortion function for a source...corresponds to finding a channel that is just right for the source and allowed distortion level.

See Chiang and Boyd (2004) for an extended discussion.

13.2 The Rate Distortion Theorem

The Shannon–McMillan theorem can be expressed as the 'zero error limit' of the rate distortion theorem, which defines a splitting criterion that identifies high probability pairs of sequences. We follow closely the treatment of Cover and Thomas (2006).

The origin of the problem is the question of representing one information source by a simpler one in such a way that the least information is lost. For example, we might have a continuous variate between 0 and 100, and wish to represent it in terms of a small set of integers in a way that minimizes the inevitable distortion that process creates. Typically, for example, an analog audio signal will be replaced by a 'digital' one. The problem is to do this in a way which least distorts the *reconstructed* audio waveform.

Suppose the original stationary, ergodic information source Y with output from a particular alphabet generates sequences of the form

$$y^n = y_1, ..., y_n.$$

These are 'digitized,' in some sense, producing a chain of 'digitized values'

$$b^n = b_1, ..., b_n,$$

where the b-alphabet is much more restricted than the y-alphabet.

b^n is, in turn, *deterministically retranslated* into a reproduction of the original signal y^n. That is, each b^m is mapped on to a unique n-length y-sequence in the alphabet of the information source Y:

$$b^m \rightarrow \hat{y}^n = \hat{y}_1, ..., \hat{y}_n.$$

Note, however, that many y^n sequences may be mapped onto the *same* retranslation sequence $\hat{y}^n$, so that information will, in general, be lost.

The central problem is to explicitly minimize that loss.

The retranslation process defines a new stationary, ergodic information source, $\hat{Y}$.

The next step is to define a *distortion measure*, $d(y, \hat{y})$, which compares the original to the retranslated path. For example the *Hamming distortion* is

$$d(y, \hat{y}) = 1, y \neq \hat{y}$$

$$d(y, \hat{y}) = 0, y = \hat{y}.$$

For continuous variates the *Squared error distortion* is

$$d(y, \hat{y}) = (y - \hat{y})^2.$$

There are many possibilities.

The distortion between paths y^n and $\hat{y}^n$ is defined as

$$d(y^n, \hat{y}^n) = \frac{1}{n} \sum_{j=1}^{n} d(y_j, \hat{y}_j). \tag{13.6}$$

Suppose that with each path y^n and b^n-path retranslation into the y-language and denoted y^n, there are associated individual, joint, and conditional probability distributions

$$p(y^n), p(\hat{y}^n), p(y^n|\hat{y}^n).$$

The *average distortion* is defined as

$$D = \sum_{y^n} p(y^n) d(y^n, \hat{y}^n). \tag{13.7}$$

It is possible, using the distributions given above, to define the information transmitted from the incoming Y to the outgoing $\hat{Y}$ process in the usual manner, using the Shannon source uncertainty of the strings:

$$I(Y, \hat{Y}) \equiv H(Y) - H(Y|\hat{Y}) = H(Y) + H(\hat{Y}) - H(Y, \hat{Y}).$$

If there is no uncertainty in Y given the retranslation $\hat{Y}$, then no information is lost. In general, this will not be true.

The *information rate distortion function* $R(D)$ for a source Y with a distortion measure $d(y, \hat{y})$ is defined as

$$R(D) = \min_{p(y,\hat{y}); \sum_{(y,\hat{y})} p(y)p(y|\hat{y})d(y,\hat{y}) \leq D} I(Y, \hat{Y}). \tag{13.8}$$

The minimization is over all conditional distributions $p(y|\hat{y})$ for which the joint distribution $p(y, \hat{y}) = p(y)p(y|\hat{y})$ satisfies the average distortion constraint (i.e., average distortion $\leq D$).

The *rate distortion theorem* states that $R(D)$ *is the maximum achievable rate of information transmission which does not exceed the distortion D*. Cover and Thomas (2006) provide details. Another interpretation is that $R(D)$ is the minimum necessary available channel capacity so that average distortion is $\leq D$.

Note that pairs of sequences $(y^n, \hat{y}^n)$ can be defined as *distortion typical*; that is, for a given average distortion D, defined in terms of a particular measure, pairs of sequences can be divided into two sets, a high probability one containing a relatively small number of (matched) pairs with $d(y^n, \hat{y}^n) \leq D$, and a low probability one containing most pairs. As $n \to \infty$, the smaller set approaches unit probability, and, for those pairs,

$$p(y^n) \geq p(\hat{y}^n|y^n) \exp[-nI(Y, \hat{Y})]. \qquad (13.9)$$

Thus, roughly speaking, $I(Y, \hat{Y})$ embodies the splitting criterion between high and low probability pairs of paths.

For the theory of interacting information sources, then, $I(Y, \hat{Y})$ can play the role of H in the dynamic 'Onsager' treatments above.

The rate distortion function can actually be calculated in many cases by using a Lagrange multiplier method – see Cover and Thomas (2006).

For a Gaussian channel having noise with variance σ^2 and zero mean, using the squared distortion measure gives

$$R(D) = 1/2 \log[\sigma^2/D], D \leq \sigma^2,$$

$$R(D) = 0, D > \sigma^2.$$

13.3   Stochastic Differential Equations

Martingales

Suppose a player in a game of chance begins with an initial fortune of some given amount, and bets $n = 1, 2, \ldots$ times according to a stochastic process in which a stochastic variable $\mathbf{X}_n$, representing the size of the player's fortune at play n, takes values $\mathbf{X}_n = x_{n,i}$ with probabilities $P_{n,i}$ such that $\sum_i P_{n,i} = 1$, where i represents a particular outcome at step n.

Assume for all n there exists a value $0 < C < \infty$ such that the expectation of $\mathbf{X}_n$,

$$E(\mathbf{X}_n) \equiv \sum_i x_{n,i} P_{n,i} < C \qquad (13.10)$$

for all n. That is, no infinite or endlessly increasing fortunes are permitted.

The state $\mathbf{X}_n = 0$, having probability P_n^0, i.e., the loss of all a player's funds, terminates the game.

We suppose it possible to define conditional probabilities at step $n + 1$ depending on the way in which the value of $\mathbf{X}_n$ was reached, so that the conditional expectation of $\mathbf{X}_{n+1}$ becomes

$$E(\mathbf{X}_{n+1}|\mathbf{X}_1, \mathbf{X}_2, ...\mathbf{X}_n) \equiv E(\mathbf{X}_{n+1}|n).$$

The 'sample space' for the probabilities defining this conditional expectation is the set of different possible sequences of the $x_{m,i} > 0$: $x_{1,i}, x_{2,j}, x_{3,k}...x_{n,q}$

Call the sequence of stochastic variables $\mathbf{X}_n$ defining the game a *Submartingale* if, at each step n,

$$E(\mathbf{X}_{n+1}|n) \geq \mathbf{X}_n,$$

a *Martingale* if

$$E(\mathbf{X}_{n+1}|n) = \mathbf{X}_n,$$

and a *Supermartingale* if

$$E(\mathbf{X}_{n+1}|n) \leq \mathbf{X}_n.$$

$\mathbf{X}_n$ is, remember, the player's fortune at step n.

Clearly a submartingale is favorable to the player, a martingale is an absolutely fair game, and a supermartingale is favorable to the house.

Regardless of the complexity of the game, the details of the playing instruments, the ways of determining gains or loss or their amounts, or any other structural factors of the underlying stochastic process, the essential content of the Martingale limit theorem is that in all three cases the sequence of stochastic variables $\mathbf{X}_n$ converges in probability 'almost everywhere' to a well-defined stochastic variable $\mathbf{X}$ as $n \to \infty$. That is, for each kind of martingale, no matter the actual sequence of winnings $x_{1,i}, x_{2,j}, ...x_{n,k}, x_{n+1,m}, ...$, you get to the same limiting stochastic variable $\mathbf{X}$. Sequences for which this does not happen have zero probability.

A simple proof of this result (Petersen, 1995) runs to several pages of dense mathematics using modern theories of abstract integration on sets. Indeed, all the asymptotic theorems we have cited require more or less arduous application of measure theory and Lebesgue integration, topics which are themselves relatively straightforward, elegant and worth study (Rudin, 1976, Royden, 1968). Proofs using more elementary approaches (Karlin and Taylor, 1975, Ch. 6) run to full chapters.

Nested Martingales

Now consider compound stochastic processes. Traditionally the simplest takes the compound game as a subset of the original:

$$\mathbf{X}_{n+1} = \mathbf{X}_n + \mathbf{A}_n(\mathbf{Y}_{n+1} - \mathbf{Y}_n). \tag{13.11}$$

Assume the filter $\mathbf{A}_n \geq 0$ is a non-negative stochastic variable, which can indeed take the value 0. This may, for example, be greater than zero only one time in ten or a hundred, on average. Taking the conditional expectation gives

$$E(\mathbf{X}_{n+1}|n) = \mathbf{X}_n + \mathbf{A}_n(E(\mathbf{Y}_{n+1}|n) - \mathbf{Y}_n) \tag{13.12}$$

where the conditional expectation of any variate $\mathbf{Z}_n$ at step n is just its value.

Since $\mathbf{A}_n \geq 0$, *the game described by the attenuated sequence* $\mathbf{X}_n$ *has the same martingale classification as does the nested game described by* $\mathbf{Y}_n$.

The Martingale transform

The X-processes in Eq. (13.11) is the *Martingale transform* of $\mathbf{Y}_n$ (Taylor, 1996, p. 232; Billingsley, 1968, p. 412), and the result is classic, representing the *impossibility of a successful betting system*.

Note that the basic Martingale transform can be rewritten as

$$\frac{\mathbf{X}_{n+1} - \mathbf{X}_n}{\mathbf{Y}_{n+1} - \mathbf{Y}_n} \equiv \frac{\Delta\mathbf{X}_n}{\Delta\mathbf{Y}_n} = \mathbf{A}_n, \tag{13.13}$$

or

$$\Delta\mathbf{X}_n = \mathbf{A}_n\Delta\mathbf{Y}_n. \tag{13.14}$$

Induction gives

$$\mathbf{X}_{n+1} = \mathbf{X}_0 + \sum_{j=1}^{n} \mathbf{A}_j\Delta\mathbf{Y}_j. \tag{13.15}$$

This notation is suggestive. In fact, the Martingale transform is the discrete analog of Ito's stochastic integral relative to a sequence of stopping times (Taylor, 1996, p. 232; Protter, 1990, p. 44; Ikeda and Watanabe, 1989, p. 48). In the stochastic integral context, the Y-process is called the 'integrator' and the A-process the 'integrand'. Further development leads toward generalizations of Brownian motion, the Poisson process, and so on (Meyer, 1989; Protter, 1990).

The basic picture is of the transmission of a signal, $\mathbf{Y}_n$, in the presence of noise, $\mathbf{A}_n$.

Stochastic differential equations

A more realistic extension of the elementary denumerable Martingale transform for our purposes is

$$\mathbf{X}_{n+1} = \mathbf{X}_n + (\mathbf{B}_{n+1} - \mathbf{B}_n)\mathbf{X}_n + \mathbf{A}_n(\mathbf{Y}_{n+1} - \mathbf{Y}_n),   \tag{13.16}$$

where $\mathbf{B}_n$ is another stochastic variable.

Using the more suggestive notation of Eqs. (13.13) and (13.14) this becomes the fundamental stochastic differential equation

$$\Delta \mathbf{X}_n = \mathbf{X}_n \Delta \mathbf{B}_n + \mathbf{A}_n \Delta \mathbf{Y}_n.   \tag{13.17}$$

Taking conditional expectations gives

$$E(\mathbf{X}_{n+1}|n) - \mathbf{X}_n =$$
$$\mathbf{X}_n(E(\mathbf{B}_{n+1}|n) - \mathbf{B}_n) + \mathbf{A}_n(E(\mathbf{Y}_{n+1}|n) - \mathbf{Y}_n).   \tag{13.18}$$

If $\mathbf{X}_n, \mathbf{A}_n \geq 0$, the martingale classification of $\mathbf{X}$ depends on those of $\mathbf{B}$ and $\mathbf{Y}$.

Extending the argument to a hierarchically linked network is straightforward, leading to the Ito stochastic integral

$$\mathbf{X}_{n+1} \approx \mathbf{X}_0 + \sum_{k=1}^{n} \mathbf{A}_k \Delta \mathbf{Y}_k.   \tag{13.19}$$

The complete hierarchical system then undergoes an iterative Z-process defined by the integrator $\mathbf{X}_j$:

$$\mathbf{Z}_{m+1} \approx \mathbf{Z}_0 + \sum_{j=1}^{m} \mathbf{C}_j \Delta \mathbf{X}_j.   \tag{13.20}$$

Extension of this development to intermediate times is complicated and involves taking the continuous limit of the Riemann-type sums of Eqs. (13.14), (13.18) and (13.19). This produces the stochastic differential equation

$$d\mathbf{X}_t = \mathbf{X}_t d\mathbf{B}_t + \mathbf{A}_t d\mathbf{Y}_t   \tag{13.21}$$

whose solution depends critically on the behavior of the second-order step-by-step 'quadratic variation', a variance-like limit of the stochastic processes. Letting $\mathbf{U}_n, \mathbf{V}_n$ be two arbitrary processes with $\mathbf{U}_0 = \mathbf{V}_0 = 0$, their quadratic variation is

$$[\mathbf{U}_n, \mathbf{V}_n] \equiv \sum_{j=1}^{n-1} (\mathbf{U}_{j+1} - \mathbf{U}_j)(\mathbf{V}_{j+1} - \mathbf{V}_j).   \tag{13.22}$$

Taking the 'infinitesimal limit' of continuous time, a term-by-term expansion of this sum can be shown to give (e.g., Meyer, 1989; Protter, 1990)

$$[\mathbf{U}_t, \mathbf{V}_t] = \mathbf{U}_t\mathbf{V}_t - \int_0^t \mathbf{U}_s d\mathbf{V}_s - \int_0^t \mathbf{V}_r d\mathbf{U}_r . \tag{13.23}$$

To put this in some perspective, classical Brownian motion has the 'structure equation' $[\mathbf{X}_t, \mathbf{X}_t] = t$. That is, for Brownian motion the jump-by-jump quadratic variation increases linearly with time. While much of the contemporary theory of financial markets is based on Brownian analogs, real processes are likely to be more complex, subject to sudden, massive, discontinuous 'phase changes' which cannot be simply characterized as diffusional.

The solution of Eq. (13.21) is a classic result in the theory of stochastic differential equations (Protter, 1990). We assume for simplicity no discontinuous jumps, and first study the 'exponential' equation

$$d\mathbf{X}_t = \mathbf{X}_t d\mathbf{B}_t \Rightarrow$$
$$\mathbf{X}_t = \mathbf{X}_0 + \int_0^t \mathbf{X}_s d\mathbf{B}_s . \tag{13.24}$$

Following Protter (1990, p. 78), this has the solution

$$\mathbf{X}_t = \epsilon(\mathbf{B})_t = \mathbf{X}_0 \exp(\mathbf{B}_t - 1/2[\mathbf{B}_t, \mathbf{B}_t]) . \tag{13.25}$$

Next, define

$$\mathbf{H}_t \equiv \int_0^t \mathbf{A}_s d\mathbf{Y}_s . \tag{13.26}$$

Equation (13.21) can be restated as

$$\mathbf{X}_t = \mathbf{H}_t + \mathbf{X}_0 + \int_0^t \mathbf{X}_s d\mathbf{B}_s . \tag{13.27}$$

For the continuous case, this has the formal solution (Protter, 1990, p. 266)

$$\epsilon_{\mathbf{H}}(\mathbf{B})_t = \epsilon(\mathbf{B})_t[\mathbf{H}_0 + \int_0^t 1/\epsilon(\mathbf{B})_s d(\mathbf{H}_s - [\mathbf{H}, \mathbf{B}]_s)] , \tag{13.28}$$

with

$$1/\epsilon(\mathbf{B}) = \epsilon(-\mathbf{B} + [\mathbf{B}, \mathbf{B}]) . \tag{13.29}$$

The structure equations defining $[\mathbf{B}, \mathbf{B}]$ and $[\mathbf{H}, \mathbf{B}]$ are critical in determining transient behavior, but not likely to have simple Brownian form.

13.4 Morse Theory

Morse theory examines relations between analytic behavior of a function – the location and character of its critical points – and the underlying topology of the manifold on which the function is defined. We are interested in a number of such functions, for example information source uncertainty on a parameter space and 'second order' iterations involving parameter manifolds determining critical behavior, for example sudden onset of a giant component in the mean number model of Chapter 2, and universality class tuning in the mean field model of Wallace (2005). These can be reformulated from a Morse theory perspective. Here we follow closely the elegant treatments of Kastner (2006) and Pettini (2007).

The essential idea of Morse theory is to examine an n-dimensional manifold M as decomposed into level sets of some function $f : M \to \mathbf{R}$ where $\mathbf{R}$ is the set of real numbers. The a-level set of f is defined as

$$f^{-1}(a) = \{x \in M : f(x) = a\},$$

the set of all points in M with $f(x) = a$. If M is compact, then the whole manifold can be decomposed into such slices in a canonical fashion between two limits, defined by the minimum and maximum of f on M. Let the part of M below a be defined as

$$M_a = f^{-1}(-\infty, a] = \{x \in M : f(x) \le a\}.$$

These sets describe the whole manifold as a varies between the minimum and maximum of f.

Morse functions are defined as a particular set of smooth functions $f : M \to \mathbf{R}$ as follows. Suppose a function f has a critical point x_c, so that the derivative $df(x_c) = 0$, with critical value $f(x_c)$. Then, f is a Morse function if its critical points are nondegenerate in the sense that the Hessian matrix of second derivatives at x_c, whose elements, in terms of local coordinates are

$$\mathcal{H}_{i,j} = \partial^2 f / \partial x^i \partial x^j,$$

has rank n, which means that it has only nonzero eigenvalues, so that there are no lines or surfaces of critical points and, ultimately, critical points are isolated.

The index of the critical point is the number of negative eigenvalues of $\mathcal{H}$ at x_c.

A level set $f^{-1}(a)$ of f is called a critical level if a is a critical value of f, that is, if there is at least one critical point $x_c \in f^{-1}(a)$.

Again following Pettini (2007), the essential results of Morse theory are:

1. If an interval $[a, b]$ contains no critical values of f, then the topology of $f^{-1}[a, v]$ does not change for any $v \in (a, b)$. Importantly, the result is valid even if f is not a Morse function, but only a smooth function.

2. If the interval $[a, b]$ contains critical values, the topology of $f^{-1}[a, v]$ changes in a manner determined by the properties of the matrix H at the critical points.

3. If $f : M \to \mathbf{R}$ is a Morse function, the set of all the critical points of f is a discrete subset of M, i.e., critical points are isolated. This is Sard's theorem.

4. If $f : M \to \mathbf{R}$ is a Morse function, with M compact, then on a finite interval $[a, b] \subset \mathbf{R}$, there is only a finite number of critical points p of f such that $f(p) \in [a, b]$. The set of critical values of f is a discrete set of $\mathbf{R}$.

5. For any differentiable manifold M, the set of Morse functions on M is an open dense set in the set of real functions of M of differentiability class r for $0 \leq r \leq \infty$.

6. Some topological invariants of M, that is, quantities that are the same for all the manifolds that have the same topology as M, can be estimated and sometimes computed exactly once all the critical points of f are known: let the Morse numbers $\mu_i (i = 0, ..., m)$ of a function f on M be the number of critical points of f of index i, (the number of negative eigenvalues of H). The Euler characteristic of the complicated manifold M can be expressed as the alternating sum of the Morse numbers of any Morse function on M,

$$\chi = \sum_{i=1}^{m} (-1)^i \mu_i.$$

The Euler characteristic reduces, in the case of a simple polyhedron, to

$$\chi = V - E + F$$

where V, E, and F are the numbers of vertices, edges, and faces in the polyhedron.

7. Another important theorem states that, if the interval $[a, b]$ contains a critical value of f with a single critical point x_c, then the topology of the set M_b defined above differs from that of M_a in a way which is determined by the index, i, of the critical point. Then M_b is homeomorphic to the manifold obtained from attaching to M_a an i-handle, i.e., the direct product of an i-disk and an $(m - i)$-disk.

Again, Pettini (2007) and Matsumoto (2002) contain mathematical details and further references.

13.5   Groupoids

Basic ideas

Following Weinstein (1996) closely, a groupoid, G, is defined by a base set A upon which some mapping – a morphism – can be defined. Note that not all possible pairs of states (a_j, a_k) in the base set A can be connected by such a morphism. Those that can define the groupoid element, a morphism $g = (a_j, a_k)$ having the natural inverse $g^{-1} = (a_k, a_j)$. Given such a pairing, it is possible to define 'natural' end-point maps $\alpha(g) = a_j, \beta(g) = a_k$ from the set of morphisms G into A, and a formally associative product in the groupoid $g_1 g_2$ provided $\alpha(g_1 g_2) = \alpha(g_1), \beta(g_1 g_2) = \beta(g_2)$, and $\beta(g_1) = \alpha(g_2)$. Then, the product is defined, and associative, $(g_1 g_2) g_3 = g_1 (g_2 g_3)$.

In addition, there are natural left and right identity elements λ_g, ρ_g such that $\lambda_g g = g = g \rho_g$ (Weinstein, 1996).

An orbit of the groupoid G over A is an equivalence class for the relation $a_j \sim Ga_k$ if and only if there is a groupoid element g with $\alpha(g) = a_j$ and $\beta(g) = a_k$. Following Cannas da Silva and Weinstein (1999), we note that a groupoid is called transitive if it has just one orbit. The transitive groupoids are the building blocks of groupoids in that there is a natural decomposition of the base space of a general groupoid into orbits. Over each orbit there is a transitive groupoid, and the disjoint union of these transitive groupoids is the original groupoid. Conversely, the disjoint union of groupoids is itself a groupoid.

The isotropy group of $a \in X$ consists of those g in G with $\alpha(g) = a = \beta(g)$. These groups prove fundamental to classifying groupoids.

If G is any groupoid over A, the map $(\alpha, \beta) : G \to A \times A$ is a morphism from G to the pair groupoid of A. The image of (α, β) is the orbit equivalence relation $\sim G$, and the functional kernel is the union of the isotropy groups. If $f : X \to Y$ is a function, then the kernel of f, $ker(f) = [(x_1, x_2) \in X \times X : f(x_1) = f(x_2)]$ defines an equivalence relation.

Groupoids may have additional structure. As Weinstein (1996) explains, a groupoid G is a topological groupoid over a base space X if G and X are topological spaces and α, β and multiplication are continuous maps. A criticism sometimes applied to groupoid theory is that their classification up to isomorphism is nothing other than the classification of equivalence relations via the orbit equivalence relation and groups via the isotropy groups. The imposition of a compatible topological structure produces a nontrivial interaction between the two structures. Above, we have introduced a metric structure on manifolds of related information sources, producing such interaction.

In essence, a groupoid is a category in which all morphisms have an inverse, here defined in terms of connection to a base point by a meaningful path of an information source dual to a cognitive process.

As Weinstein (1996) points out, the morphism (α, β) suggests another way of looking at groupoids. A groupoid over A identifies not only which elements of A are equivalent to one another (isomorphic), but *it also parametizes the different ways (isomorphisms) in which two elements can be equivalent*, i.e., in our context, all possible information sources dual to some cognitive process. Given the information theoretic characterization of cognition presented above, this produces a full modular cognitive network in a highly natural manner.

Brown (1987) describes the fundamental structure as follows:

A groupoid should be thought of as a group with many objects, or with many identities... A groupoid with one object is essentially just a group. So the notion of groupoid is an extension of that of groups. It gives an additional convenience, flexibility and range of applications...

EXAMPLE 1. A disjoint union [of groups] $G = \cup_\lambda G_\lambda, \lambda \in \Lambda$, is a groupoid: the product ab is defined if and only if a, b belong to the same G_λ, and ab is then just the product in the group G_λ. There is an identity 1_λ for each $\lambda \in \Lambda$. The maps α, β coincide and map G_λ to $\lambda, \lambda \in \Lambda$.

EXAMPLE 2. An equivalence relation R on [a set] X becomes a groupoid with $\alpha, \beta : R \to X$ the two projections, and product $(x, y)(y, z) = (x, z)$ whenever $(x, y), (y, z) \in R$. There is an identity, namely (x, x), for each $x \in X$...

Weinstein (1996) makes the following fundamental point:

Almost every interesting equivalence relation on a space B arises in a natural way as the orbit equivalence relation of some groupoid G over B. Instead of dealing directly with the orbit space B/G as an object in the category S_{map} of sets and mappings, one should consider instead the groupoid G itself as an object in the category G_{htp} of groupoids and homotopy classes of morphisms.

The groupoid approach has become quite popular in the study of networks of coupled dynamical systems which can be defined by differential equation models, (e.g., Golubitsky and Stewart 2006).

Global and local symmetry groupoids

Here we follow Weinstein (1996), using his example of a finite tiling. Consider a tiling of the Euclidean plane R^2 by identical 2 by 1 rectangles, specified by the set X (one-dimensional) where the grout between tiles is $X = H \cup V$, having $H = R \times Z$ and $V = 2Z \times R$, where R is the set of real numbers and Z the integers. Call each connected component of $R^2 \backslash X$, that is, the complement of the two dimensional real plane intersecting X, a tile.

Let Γ be the group of those rigid motions of R^2 which leave X invariant, i.e., the normal subgroup of translations by elements of the lattice $\Lambda = H \cap V = 2Z \times Z$ (corresponding to corner points of the tiles), together with reflections through each of the points $1/2\Lambda = Z \times 1/2Z$, and across the horizontal and vertical lines through those points. As noted by Weinstein (1996), much is lost in this coarse-graining, in particular the same symmetry group would arise if we replaced X entirely by the lattice Λ of corner points. Γ retains no information about the local structure of the tiled plane. In the case of a real tiling, restricted to the finite set $B = [0, 2m] \times [0, n]$ the symmetry group shrinks drastically: the subgroup leaving $X \cap B$ invariant contains just four elements even though a repetitive pattern is clearly visible. A two-stage groupoid approach recovers the lost structure.

We define the transformation groupoid of the action of Γ on R^2 to be the set

$$G(\Gamma, R^2) = \{(x, \gamma, y | x \in R^2, y \in R^2, \gamma \in \Gamma, x = \gamma y\},$$

with the partially defined binary operation

$$(x, \gamma, y)(y, \nu, z) = (x, \gamma\nu, z).$$

Here, $\alpha(x, \gamma, y) = x$, and $\beta(x, \gamma, y) = y$, and the inverses are natural.

We can form the restriction of G to B (or any other subset of R^2) by defining

$$G(\Gamma, R^2)|_B = \{g \in G(\Gamma, R^2) | \alpha(g), \beta(g) \in B\}.$$

1. An orbit of the groupoid G over B is an equivalence class for the relation $x \sim_G y$ if and only if there is a groupoid element g with $\alpha(g) = x$ and $\beta(g) = y$. Two points are in the same orbit if they are similarly placed within their tiles or within the grout pattern.

2. The isotropy group of $x \in B$ consists of those g in G with $\alpha(g) = x = \beta(g)$. It is trivial for every point except those in $1/2\Lambda \cap B$, for which it is $Z_2 \times Z_2$, the direct product of integers modulo two with itself.

By contrast, embedding the tiled structure within a larger context permits definition of a much richer structure, i.e., the identification of local symmetries.

We construct a second groupoid as follows. Consider the plane R^2 as being decomposed as the disjoint union of $P_1 = B \cap X$ (the grout), $P_2 = B \backslash P_1$ (the complement of P_1 in B, which is the tiles), and $P_3 = R^2 \backslash B$ (the exterior of the tiled room). Let E be the group of all Euclidean motions of the plane, and define the local symmetry groupoid G_{loc} as the set of triples (x, γ, y) in $B \times E \times B$ for which $x = \gamma y$, and for which y has a neighborhood $\mathcal{U}$ in R^2 such that $\gamma(\mathcal{U} \cap P_i) \subseteq P_i$ for $i = 1, 2, 3$. The composition is given by the same formula as for $G(\Gamma, R^2)$.

For this groupoid-in-context there are only a finite number of orbits:

$\mathcal{O}_1 = $ interior points of the tiles.

$\mathcal{O}_2 = $ interior edges of the tiles.

$\mathcal{O}_3 = $ interior crossing points of the grout.

$\mathcal{O}_4 = $ exterior boundary edge points of the tile grout.

$\mathcal{O}_5 = $ boundary 'T' points.

$\mathcal{O}_6 = $ boundary corner points.

The isotropy group structure is, however, now very rich indeed:

The isotropy group of a point in $\mathcal{O}_1$ is now isomorphic to the entire rotation group O_2.

It is $Z_2 \times Z_2$ for $\mathcal{O}_2$.

For $\mathcal{O}_3$ it is the eight-element dihedral group D_4.

For $\mathcal{O}_4, \mathcal{O}_5$ and $\mathcal{O}_6$ it is simply Z_2.

These are the 'local symmetries' of the tile-in-context.

13.6 'Biological' Renormalization

Following the classic phase transition arguments of Wilson (1971), the quantity of interest, F, and the correlation length – the degree of coherence along the embedding structure of interest – scale under renormalization clustering in chunks of size R, here taken as an appropriate topological distance measure, as

$$F[Q_R, J_R]/f(R) = F[J, Q],$$
$$\chi[Q_R, J_R]R = \chi(Q, J), \tag{13.30}$$

with $f(1) = 1, Q_1 = Q, J_1 = J$. Q is to be seen as an inverse temperature analog, and in the limit, again following the patterning of Wilson (1971), we will allow the 'external field' $J \to 0$. Other approaches are possible.

Differentiating these two equations with respect to R, so that the right hand sides are zero, and solving for dQ_R/dR and dJ_R/dR gives, after some consolidation, expressions of the form

$$dQ_R/dR = u_1 d\log(f)/dR + u_2/R,$$
$$dJ_R/dR = v_1 J_R d\log(f)/dR + \frac{v_2}{R} J_R. \tag{13.31}$$

The $u_i, v_i, i = 1, 2$ are functions of Q_R, J_R, but not explicitly of R itself.

We expand these equations about the *critical value* $Q_R = Q_C$ and about $J_R = 0$, obtaining

$$dQ_R/dR = (Q_R - Q_C)yd\log(f)/dR + (Q_R - Q_C)z/R,$$
$$dJ_R/dR = wJ_R d\log(f)/dR + xJ_R/R. \tag{13.32}$$

The terms $y = du_1/dQ_R|_{Q_R=Q_C}, z = du_2/dQ_R|_{Q_R=Q_C}, w = v_1(Q_C, 0), x = v_2(Q_C, 0)$ are constants.

Solving the first of these equations gives

$$Q_R = Q_C + (Q - Q_C)R^z f(R)^y, \tag{13.33}$$

again remembering that $Q_1 = Q, J_1 = J, f(1) = 1$.

Wilson's essential trick is to iterate on this relation, which is supposed to converge rapidly near the critical point (Binney et al., 1992), assuming that for Q_R near Q_C, we have

$$Q_C/2 \approx Q_C + (Q - Q_C)R^z f(R)^y. \tag{13.34}$$

We iterate in two steps, first solving this for $f(R)$ in terms of known values, and then solving for R, finding a value R_C that we then substitute into the first of Eqs. (13.32) to obtain an expression for $H[Q, 0]$ in terms of known functions and parameter values.

The first step gives the general result

$$f(R_C) \approx \frac{[Q_C/(Q_C - Q)]^{1/y}}{2^{1/y} R_C^{z/y}}. \tag{13.35}$$

Solving this for R_C and substituting into the first expression of Eq. (13.30) gives, as a first iteration of a far more general procedure (Shirkov and Kovalev, 2001), the result

$$F[Q, 0] \approx \frac{F[Q_C/2, 0]}{f(R_C)} = \frac{F_0}{f(R_C)},$$
$$\chi(Q, 0) \approx \chi(Q_C/2, 0)R_C = \chi_0 R_C, \tag{13.36}$$

which are the essential relationships.

Note that a power law of the form $f(R) = R^m, m = 3$, which is the direct physical analog, may not be biologically reasonable, since it says that F can grow very rapidly as a function of increased substrait size. Such rapid growth is not necessarily observed.

Taking the biologically realistic example of non-integral 'fractal' exponential growth,

$$f(R) = R^\delta,\tag{13.37}$$

where $\delta > 0$ is a real number which may be quite small. Eq. (13.35) can be solved for R_C, obtaining

$$R_C = \frac{[Q_C/(Q_C - Q)]^{[1/(\delta y + z)]}}{2^{1/(\delta y + z)}}\tag{13.38}$$

for Q near Q_C. Note that, for a given value of y, one might characterize the relation $\alpha \equiv \delta y + z = \text{constant}$ as a 'tunable universality class relation' in the sense of Albert and Barabasi (2002).

Substituting this value for R_C back into Eq. (13.35) gives a complex expression for F, having three parameters: δ, y, z.

A more biologically interesting choice for $f(R)$ is a logarithmic curve that 'tops out', for example

$$f(R) = m \log(R) + 1.\tag{13.39}$$

Again $f(1) = 1$.

Using Mathematica 4.2 or above to solve Eq. (13.35) for R_C gives

$$R_C = [\frac{S}{LambertW[S \exp(z/my)]}]^{y/z},\tag{13.40}$$

where

$$S \equiv (z/my)2^{-1/y}[Q_C/(Q_C - Q)]^{1/y}.$$

The transcendental function LambertW(x) is defined by the relation

$$LambertW(x) \exp(LambertW(x)) = x.$$

It arises in the theory of random networks and in renormalization strategies for quantum field theories.

An asymptotic relation for $f(R)$ would be of particular biological interest, implying that F increases to a limiting value with population growth. Such a pattern is broadly consistent with, for example, calculations of the degree of allelic heterozygosity as a function of population size under a balance between genetic drift and neutral mutation (Hartl and Clark, 1997; Ridley, 1996). Taking

$$f(R) = \exp[m(R - 1)/R]\tag{13.41}$$

gives a system which begins at 1 when $R = 1$, and approaches the asymptotic limit $\exp(m)$ as $R \to \infty$. Mathematica 4.2 finds

$$R_C = \frac{my/z}{LambertW[A]}, \quad (13.42)$$

where

$$A \equiv (my/z)\exp(my/z)[2^{1/y}[Q_C/(Q_C - Q)]^{-1/y}]^{y/z}.$$

These developments indicate the possibility of taking the theory significantly beyond arguments by abduction from simple physical models, although the notorious difficulty of implementing information theory existence arguments will undoubtedly persist.

Universality class

Physical systems undergoing phase transition usually have relatively pure renormalization properties, with quite different systems clumped into the same 'universality class', having fixed exponents at transition (Binney et al., 1992). Biological phenomena may be far more complicated. If the system of interest is a mix of subgroups with different values of some significant renormalization parameter m in the expression for $f(R,m)$, according to a distribution $\rho(m)$, then, at least to first order,

$$F[Q_R, J_R] = < f(R,m) > F[Q,J] \equiv F[Q,J] \int f(R,m)\rho(m)dm. \quad (13.43)$$

If $f(R) = 1 + m\log(R)$ then, given any distribution for m,

$$< f(R) >= 1+ < m > \log(R), \quad (13.44)$$

where $< m >$ is simply the mean of m over that distribution.

Other forms of $f(R)$ having more complicated dependencies on the distributed parameter or parameters, like the power law R^δ, do not produce such a simple result. Taking $\rho(\delta)$ as a normal distribution, for example, gives

$$< R^\delta >= R^{<\delta>} \exp[(1/2)(\log(R^\sigma))^2], \quad (13.45)$$

where σ^2 is the distribution variance. The renormalization properties of this function can be determined from Eq. (13.30).

Thus the phase transition properties of mixed systems will not in general be simply related to those of a single subcomponent, a matter of possible empirical importance: if sets of relevant parameters defining renormalization universality classes are indeed distributed, experiments observing pure phase changes may be very difficult. Tuning among different possible renormalization strategies in response to external signals would result in even greater ambiguity in recognizing and classifying biological phase transitions.

Important aspects of mechanism may be reflected in the combination of renormalization properties and the details of their distribution across subsystems.

In sum, biological systems are likely to have very rich patterns of phase transition that may not display the simplistic, indeed, literally elemental, purity familiar to physicists. Overall mechanisms will, however, still remain significantly constrained by the theory, in the general sense of probability limit theorems.

The more biologically realistic renormalization strategies given above produce sets of several parameters defining the universality class.

Suppose, now, that the renormalization properties of a system at some 'time' k are characterized by a set of (possibly coarse-grained) parameters $A_k \equiv \alpha_1^k, ..., \alpha_m^k$. Fixed parameter values define a particular universality class for the renormalization. We suppose that, over a sequence of 'times', the universality class properties can be characterized by a path $x_n = A_0, A_1, ..., A_{n-1}$ having significant serial correlations which, in fact, permit definition of an adiabatically piecewise stationary ergodic information source associated with the paths x_n. We call that source **X**.

Suppose also that the set of impinging signals is also highly structured and forms another information source **Y** that interacts not only with the system of interest globally, but specifically with its universality class properties as characterized by **X**. **Y** is necessarily associated with a set of paths y_n.

Pair the two sets of paths into a joint path, $z_n \equiv (x_n, y_y)$ and invoke an inverse coupling parameter, Q, between the information sources and their paths. This leads, by the arguments above, to phase transition punctuation of $I[Q]$, the mutual information between **X** and **Y**, under either the joint asymptotic equipartition theorem or under limitation by a distortion measure, through the rate distortion theorem. The essential point is that $I[Q]$ is a splitting criterion under these theorems, and thus partakes of the homology with free energy density.

Activation of universality class tuning then becomes itself a punctuated event in response to increasing linkage between the biological structure of interest and an external structured signal or some particular system of internal events.

This iterated argument exactly parallels the extension of the general linear model to the hierarchical linear model in regression theory (Byrk and Raudenbusch, 2001).

13.7 Large Deviations

It is of some interest to more explicitly carry through the program suggested by Campagnat *et al.* (2006) via a recapitulation of large deviations and fluctuation formalism.

Information source uncertainty, according to the Shannon–McMillan theorem, serves as a splitting criterion between high and low probability sequences (or pairs of them) and displays the fundamental characteristic of a growing body of work in applied probability often termed the large deviations program (LDP). This seeks to unite information theory, statistical mechanics, and the theory of fluctuations under a single umbrella.

Following Dembo and Zeitouni, (1998, p. 2), let $X_1, X_2, ... X_n$ be a sequence of independent, standard Normal, real-valued random variables and let

$$S_n = \frac{1}{n} \sum_{j=1}^{n} X_j .$$

(13.46)

Since S_n is again a Normal random variable with zero mean and variance $1/n$, for all $\delta > 0$

$$\lim_{n \to \infty} P(|S_n| \geq \delta) = 0 ,$$

(13.47)

where P is the probability that the absolute value of S_n is greater or equal to δ. Some manipulation, however, gives

$$P(|S_n| \geq \delta) = 1 - \frac{1}{\sqrt{2\pi}} \int_{-\delta\sqrt{n}}^{\delta\sqrt{n}} \exp(-x^2/2) dx ,$$

(13.48)

so that

$$\lim_{n \to \infty} \frac{\log P(|S_n| \geq \delta)}{n} = -\delta^2/2 .$$

(13.49)

This can be rewritten for large n as

$$P(|S_n| \geq \delta) \approx \exp(-n\delta^2/2) .$$

(13.50)

That is, for large n, the probability of a large deviation in S_n follows something much like the asymptotic equipartition relation of the Shannon–McMillan theorem, so that meaningful paths of length n all have approximately the same probability $P(n) \propto \exp(-nH[\mathbf{X}])$.

Questions about meaningful paths appear suddenly as formally isomorphic to the central argument of the LDP which encompasses statistical mechanics, fluctuation theory, and information theory into a single structure (Dembo and Zeitouni, 1998).

Again, the cardinal tenet of large deviation theory is that the rate function $-\delta^2/2$ can, under proper circumstances, be expressed as a mathematical entropy having the standard form

$$-\sum_k p_k \log p_k , \tag{13.51}$$

for some set of probabilities p_k.

Next, we briefly recapitulate part of the standard treatment of large fluctuations (e.g., Onsager and Machlup, 1953; Fredlin and Wentzell, 1998).

The macroscopic behavior of a complicated physical system in time is assumed to be described by the phenomenological Onsager relations giving large-scale fluxes as

$$\sum_i C_{i,j} dK_j/dt = \partial S/\partial K_i , \tag{13.52}$$

where the $C_{i,j}$ are appropriate constants, S is the system entropy, and the K_i are the generalized coordinates which parametize the system's free energy.

Entropy is defined from free energy F by a Legendre transform – more of which follows below:

$$S \equiv F - \sum_j K_j \partial F/\partial K_j,$$

where the K_j are appropriate system parameters.

Neglecting volume problems for the moment, free energy can be defined from the system's partition function Z as

$$F(K) = \log[Z(K)].$$

The partition function Z, in turn, is defined from the system Hamiltonian – defining the energy states – as

$$Z(K) = \sum_j \exp[-KE_j],$$

where K is an inverse temperature or other parameter and the E_j are the energy states.

Inverting the Onsager equation gives

$$dK_i/dt = \sum_j L_{i,j} \partial S/\partial K_j = L_i(K_1, ..., K_m, t) \equiv L_i(K, t) . \tag{13.53}$$

The terms $\partial S/\partial K_i$ are macroscopic driving forces dependent on the entropy gradient.

Let a white Brownian noise $\epsilon(t)$ perturb the system, so that

$$dK_i/dt = \sum_j L_{i,j}\partial S/\partial K_j + \epsilon(t)$$

$$= L_i(K,t) + \epsilon(t), \qquad (13.54)$$

where the time averages of ϵ are $< \epsilon(t) >= 0$ and $< \epsilon(t)\epsilon(0) >= D\delta(t)$. $\delta(t)$ is the Dirac delta function, and we take K as a vector in the K_i.

Following Luchinsky (1997), if the probability that the system starts at some initial macroscopic parameter state K_0 at time $t = 0$ and gets to the state $K(t)$ at time t is $P(K,t)$, then a somewhat subtle development (e.g., Feller, 1971) gives the forward Fokker–Planck equation for P:

$$\partial P(K,t)/\partial t = -\nabla \cdot (L(K,t)P(K,t)) + (D/2)\nabla^2 P(K,t). \qquad (13.55)$$

In the limit of weak noise intensity this can be solved using the WKB (i.e., the eikonal) approximation, as follows. Take

$$P(K,t) = z(K,t)\exp(-s(K,t)/D). \qquad (13.56)$$

$z(K,t)$ is a prefactor and $s(K,t)$ is a classical action satisfying the Hamilton–Jacobi equation, which can be solved by integrating the Hamiltonian equations of motion. The equation reexpresses $P(K,t)$ in the usual parametized negative exponential format.

Let $p \equiv \nabla s$. Substituting and collecting terms of similar order in D gives

$$dK/dt = p + L,$$

$$dp/dt = -\partial L/\partial K p, \qquad (13.57)$$

and

$$-\partial s/\partial t \equiv h(K,p,t) = pL(K,t) + \frac{p^2}{2}, \qquad (13.58)$$

with $h(K,t)$ the Hamiltonian for appropriate boundary conditions.

Again, following Luchinsky (1997), these Hamiltonian equations have two different types of solution, depending on p. For $p = 0, dK/dt = L(K,t)$, describing the system in the absence of noise. We expect that with finite noise intensity the system will give rise to a distribution about this deterministic path. Solutions for which $p \neq 0$ correspond to *optimal paths* along which the system will move with overwhelming probability.

These results can, however, again be directly derived as a special case of a Large Deviation Principle based on generalized entropies mathematically similar to Shannon's uncertainty from information theory, bypassing the Hamiltonian formulation entirely.

Bibliography

Adami, C., N. Cerf, 2000, Physical complexity of symbolic sequences, Physica D, 137:62–69.

Adami, C., Ofria, T. Collier, 2000, Evolution of biological complexity, Proceedings of the National Academy of Sciences, 97:4463–4468.

Albert, R., A. Barabasi, 2002, Statistical mechanics of complex networks, Reviews of Modern Physics, 74:47–97.

Alzheimer's Association, 2006, African-Americans and Alzheimer's disease: the silent epidemic. www.alz.org.

Andre, I., C. Strauss, D. Kaplan, P. Bradley, D. Baker, 2008, Emergence of symmetry in homooligomeric biological assemblies, Proceedings of the National Academy of Sciences, 105:16148–16152.

Anfinsen, C., 1973, Principles that govern the folding of protein chains, Science, 181:223–230.

Arnett, J., 2008, The neglected 95%, The American Psychologist, 63:602–614.

Ash, R., 1990, Information Theory, Dover, New York.

Atiyah, M., I. Singer, 1963, The index of elliptical operators on compact manifolds, Bulletin of the American Mathematical Society, 69:322–433.

Atlan, H., I. Cohen, 1998, Immune information, self organization, and meaning, International Immunology, 10:711–717.

Atmanspacher, H., 2006, Toward an information theoretical implementation of contextual conditions for consciousness, Acta Biotheoretica, 54:157–160.

Avital, E., E. Jablonka, 2000, Animal Traditions: Behavioral Inheritance in Evolution, Cambridge University Press, New York.

Baars, B., 1988, A Cognitive Theory of Consciousness, Cambridge University Press, New York.

Baars, B., 2005, Global workspace theory of consciousness: toward a cognitive neuroscience of human experience, Progress in Brain Research, 150:45–53.

Baars, B., S. Franklin, 2003, How conscious experience and working memory interact, Trends in Cognitive Science, 7:166–172.

Backdahl, L., A. Bushell, S. Beck, 2009, Inflammatory signalling as mediator of epigenetic modulation in tissue-specific chronic inflammation, The International Journal of Biochemistry and Cell Biology, 41:176–184.

Balasubramanian, K., 1980, The symmetry groups of nonrigid molecules as generalized wreath products and their representations, Journal of Chemical Physics, 72:665–677.

Balasubramanian, K., 2004, Relativistic double group spinor representations of nonrigid molecules, Journal of Chemical Physics, 120:5524–5535.

Balazsi, G., A. van Oudenaarden, J. Collins, 2011, Cellular decision making and biological noise: from microbes to mammals, Cell, 144:910–925.

Barker, D., 2002, Fetal programming of conronary heart disease, Trends in Endocrinology and Metabolism, 13:364–372.

Barker, D., T. Forsen, A. Utela, C. Osmong, J. Erikson, 2002, Size at birth and resilience to effects of poor living conditions in adult life: longitudinal study, British Medical Journal, 323:1261–1262.

Barkow, J., L. Cosmides, J. Tooby (eds.), 1992, The Adapted Mind: Biological Approaches to Mind and Culture, University of Toronto Press, Toronto.

Bebbington, P., 1993, Transcultural aspects of affective disorders, International Review of Psychiatry, 5:145–156.

Beck, C., F. Schlogl, 1993, Thermodynamics of Chaotic Systems, Cambridge University Press, New York.

Begley, C., L. Ellis, 2012, Raise standards for preclinical cancer research, Nature, 483:531–533.

Ben-Jonathan, N., E. Hugo, T. Brandenbourg, 2009, Effects of bisphenol A on adipokine release from human adipose tissue: implications for the metabolic syndrome, Molecular Cell Endocrinology, 304:49–54.

Bennett, C., 1988, Logical depth and physical complexity. In R. Herkin (ed.), The Universal Turing Machine: A Half-Century Survey, Oxford University Press, Oxford, pp. 227–257.

Bernstein Research, 2010, The Long View - R & D Productivity, Boston.

Billingsley, P., 1968, Convergence of Probability Measures, John Wiley and Sons, New York.

Binney, J., N. Dowrick, A. Fisher, M. Newman, 1992, The Theory of Critical Phenomena, Clarendon Press, Oxford.

Bjorntorp, P., 2001, Do stress reactions cause abdominal obesity and comorbidities? Obesity Reviews, 2:73–86.

Boccaletti, S., V. Latora, Y. Moreno, M. Chavez, D. Hwang, 2006, Complex networks: structure and dynamics, Physics Reports, 424:175–208.

Bonner, J., 1980, The Evolution of Culture in Animals, Princeton University Press, Princeton.

Borkar, S., 2007, Thousand core chips – a technology perspective, DAC 2007, ACM 978-1-59593-627-1/01/0006

Bos, R., 2007, Continuous representations of groupoids, arXiv:math/0612639.

Brock, C., S. Salinsky, 1993, Empathy: an essential skill for understanding the physician-patient relationship in clinical practice, Family Medicine, 25:245–248.

Brown, G., T. Harris, J. Peto, 1973, Life events and psychiatric disorders, II: nature of causal link, Psychological Medicine, 3:159–176.

Brown, R., 1987, From groups to groupoids: a brief survey, Bulletin of the London Mathematical Society, 19:113–134.

Buneci, M., 2003, Representare de Groupoizi, Editura Mirton, Timosoara.

Burns, J., D. Job, M. Bastin, H. Whalley, T. Macgillivary, E. Johnstone, S. Lawrie, 2003, Structural disconnectivity in schizophrenia: a diffusion tensor magnetic resonance imaging study, British Journal of Psychiatry, 182:439–443.

Byers, N., 1999, E. Noether's discovery of the deep connection between symmetries and conservation laws, Israel Mathematical Conference Proceedings, Vol. 12. arXiv physics/9807044.

Byrk, A., S. Raudenbusck, 2001, Hierarchical linear models: applications and data analysis methods, Sage Publications, New York.

Cannas Da Silva, A., A.Weinstein, 1999, Geometric Models for Noncommutative Algebras, American Mathematical Society, Providence.

Caspi, A., T. Moffitt, 2002, Role of genotype in the cycle of violence in maltreated children, Science, 297:851–854.

Caspi, A., K. Sugden, T. Moffitt, 2003, Influence of life stress on depression: moderation by a polymorphism in the 5-HTT gene, Science, 301:386–389.

Caspi, A., T. Moffitt, 2006, Gene-environment interactions in psychiatry: joining forces with neuroscience, Nature Reviews Neuroscience, 7:583–590.

CDC, 2003, 1991–2001 Prevalence of Obesity Among US Adults, by Characteristics: Behavioral Risk Factor Surviellance System, Self Reported Data.

Champagnat, N., R. Ferriere, S. Meleard, 2006, Unifying evolutionary dynamics: from individual stochastic process to macroscopic models, Theoretical Population Biology, 69:297–321.

Chiang, M., S. Boyd, 2004, Geometric programming duals of channel capacity and rate distortion, IEEE Transactions on Information Theory, 50:245–255.

Chien, P., J. Weissman, 2001, Conformational diversity in a yeast prion dictates its seeding specificity, Nature, 410:223–227.

Chou, K.C., G. Maggiora, 1998, Domain structural class prediction, Protein Engineering, 11:523–528.

Clougherty, J., J. Levy, L. Kubzansky, P. Ryan, S. Suglia, M. Canner, R. Wright, 2007, Synergistic effects of traffic-related air pollution and exposure to violence on urban asthma etiology, Environmental Health Perspectives, 115:1140–1146.

Cohen, I., 1992, The cognitive principle challenges clonal selection, Immunology Today, 13:441–444.

Cohen, I., 2000, Tending Adam's Garden: Evolving the Cognitive Immune Self, Academic Press, New York.

Cohen, I., 2006, Immune system computation and the immunological homunculus. In Nierstrasz, O., J. Whittle, D. Harel, G. Reggio (eds.), MoDELS 2006, LNCS, vol. 4199, Springer, Heidelberg, pp. 499–512, .

Cohen, I., D. Harel, 2007, Explaining a complex living system: dynamics, multi-scaling, and emergence. Journal of the Royal Society: Interface, 4:175-182.

Cohen, M., A. Varki, 2010, The sialome-far more than the sum of its parts, OMICS, 14:455–464.

Coplan, J., 2005, personal communication.

Cordes, M., R. Burton, N. Walsh, C. McKnight, R. Sauer, 2000, An evolutionary bridge to a new protein fold, Nature Structural Biology, 7:1129–1132.

Courchesne, E., K. Pierce, 2005, Why the frontal cortex in autism might be talking only to itself, Current Opinion in Neurobiology, 15:225–230.

Cover, T., J. Thomas, 2006, Elements of Information Theory, Second Edition, Wiley, New York.

Cummings, R., 2009, The repertoire of glycan determinants in the human glycome, Molecular Biosystems, 5:1087–1104.

Dam, T., T. Gerken, B. Cavada, K. Nascimento, T. Moura, C.F. Brewer, 2007, Binding studies of α-GalNAc-specific lectins to the α-GalNAc(Tn-antigen) form of porcine submaxilary mucin and its smaller fragments, Journal of Biological Chemistry, 38:28256–28263.

Dam, T., C.F. Brewer, 2008, Effects of clustered epitopes in multivalent ligand-receptor interactions, Biochemistry, 47:8470–8476.

Dam, T., C.F. Brewer, 2010, Lectins as pattern recognition molecules: The effects of epitope density in innate immunity, Glycobiology, 20:270–279.

de Groot, S., P. Mazur, 1984, Non-Equilibrium Thermodynamics, Dover, New York.

Dembo, A., O. Zeitouni, 1998, Large Deviations and Applications, Springer, New York.

Diekmann U., R. Law, 1996, The dynamical theory of coevolution: a derivation from stochastic ecological processes, Journal of Mathematical Biology, 34:579–612.

Dietrich, K., R. Douglas, P. Succop, O. Berger, R. Bornschein, 2001, Early exposure to lead and juvenile delinquency, Neurotoxicology and Teratology, 23:511–518.

Dill, K., S. Banu Ozkan, T. Weikl, J. Chodera, V. Voelz, 2007, The protein folding problem: when will it be solved? Current Opinion in Structural Biology, 17:342–346.

Dobson, C., 2003, Protein folding and misfolding, Nature, 426:884–890.

Dohrenwend, B.P., B.S. Dohrenwend, 1974, Social and cultural influences on psychopathology, Annual Review of Psychology, 25:417–452.

Downing, R., K. Rickels, 1982, The impact of favorable and unfavorable life events on psychotropic drug response, Psychopharmacology, 78:97–100.

Dretske, F., 1994, The explanatory role of information, Philosophical Transactions of the Royal Society A, 349:59–70.

DSM-IV, 1994, Diagnostic and Statistical Manual, Fourth Edition, American Psychiatric Association, Washington, DC.

Durham, W., 1991, Coevolution: Genes, Culture, and Human Diversity, Stanford University Press, Palo Alto.

Eaton, W., 1978, Life events, social supports, and psychiatric symptoms: a reanalysis of the New Haven data, Journal of Health and Social Behavior, 19:230–234.

Eldredge, N., S. Gould, 1972, Punctuated equilibrium: an alternative to phyletic gradualism. In T. Schopf (ed.), Models in Paleobiology, Freeman, Cooper and Co., San Francisco, pp. 82–115.

El Gamal, A., Y. Kim, 2010, Lecture Notes on Network Information Theory, arXiv:1001.3404v4.

Ellis, R., 1985, Entropy, Large Deviations, and Statistical Mechanics, Springer, New York.

English, T., 1996, Evaluation of evolutionary and genetic optimizers: no free lunch. In Fogel, L., P. Angeline, T. Back (eds.), Evolutionary Programming V: Proceedings of the Fifth Annual Conference on Evolutionary Programming, MIT Press, Cambridge, MA, pp. 163–169.

Erdos, P., A. Renyi, 1960, On the evolution of random graphs, Magyar Tud. Akad. Mat. Kutato Int. Kozl, 5:17–61.

Ewens, W., 2004, Mathematical Population Genetics, Springer, New York.

Fanon F., 1966, The Wretched of the Earth, Evergreen Press, New York.

Feller, W., 1971, An Introduction to Probability Theory and its Applications, John Wiley and Sons, New York.

Feynman, R., 2000, Lectures on Computation, Westview Press, New York.

Fillit, H., D. Nash, T. Rundek, A. Zukerman, 2008, Cardiovascular risk factors and dementia, American Journal of Geriatric Pharmacotherapy, 6:100–118.

Fodor, J., M. Piattelli-Palmarini, 2010, What Darwin Got Wrong, Farrar, Straus, and Giroux, New York.

Foley, D., J. Craid, R. Morley, C. Olsson, T. Dwyer, K. Smith, R. Saffery, 2009, Prospects for epigenetic epidemiology, American Journal of Epidemiology, 169:389–400.

Forlenza, M., A. Baum, 2000, Psychosocial influences on cancer progression: alternative cellular and molecular mechanisms, Current Opinion in Psychiatry, 13:639–645.

Fredlin, M., A. Wentzell, 1998, Random Perturbations of Dynamical Systems, Springer, New York.

Fullilove, M., 2004, Root Shock: How Tearing Up City Neighborhoods Hurts America and What We Can Do About It, Balantine Books, New York.

Fullilove, M., R. Wallace, 2011, Serial forced displacement in American cities, 1916-2010, Journal of Urban Health, 88:381–389.

Gilbert, P., 2001, Evolutionary approaches to psychopathology: the role of natural defenses, Australian and New Zealand Journal of Psychiatry, 35:17–27.

Glass, T., K. Bandeen-Roche, M. McAtee, K. Bolla, A. Todd, B. Schwartz, 2009, Neighborhood psychosocial hazards and the association of cumulative lead dose with cognitive function in older adults, American Journal of Epidemiology, 169:683–692.

Glazebrook, J.F., R. Wallace, 2009a, Rate distortion manifolds as model spaces for cognitive information, Informatica, 33:309–346.

Glazebrook, J.F., R. Wallace, 2009b, Small worlds and red queens in the global workspace: an information-theoretic approach, Cognitive Systems Research, 10:333–365,

Gluckman, B., T. Netoff, E. Neel, W. Ditto, M. Spano, S. Schiff, 1996, Stochastic resonance in a neuronal network from mammalian brain, Physical Review Letters, 77:4098–4101.

Goldschmidt, L., P. Teng, R. Riek, D. Eisenberg, 2010, Identifying the amylome, proteins capable of forming amyloid-like fibrils, Proceedings of the National Academy of Sciences, 107:3487–3492.

Golubitsky, M., I. Stewart, 2006, Nonlinear dynamics and networks: the groupoid formalism, Bulletin of the American Mathematical Society, 43:305–364.

Gomez, J., M. Verdu, F. Perfectti, 2010, Ecological interactions are evolutionarily conserved across the entire tree of life, Nature, 465:918–921.

Goodsell, D., A. Olson, 2000, Structural symmetry and protein function, Annual Reviews of Biophysics and Biomolecular Structure, 29:105–153.

Gordon A., 2000, Cultural identity and illness: Fulani views, Culture, Medicine and Psychiatry, 24:297–330.

Gould, S., R. Lewontin, 1979, The spandrels of San Marco and the Panglossian paradigm: A critique of the adaptationist programme, Proceedings of the Royal Society of London, B, 205:581–598.

Gould, S., 2002, The Structure of Evolutionary Theory, Harvard University Press, Cambridge, MA.

Gunderson, L., 2000, Ecological resilience – in theory and application, Annual Reviews of Ecological Systematics, 31:425–439.

Gupta, G., A. Surolia, S. Sampath Kumar, 2010, Lectin microarrays for glycomic analysis, OMICS, 14:419–436.

Haataja, L., T. Gurlo, C. Huang, P. Butler, 2008, Islet amyloid in type 2 diabetes, and the toxic oligomer hypothesis, Endocrine Reviews, 29:303–316.

Haller, J., J. Halasz, 2000, Effects of two acute stressors on the anxiolytic efficacy of chlordiazepoxide, Psychopharmacology, 151:1–6.

Haller, J., 2001, The link between stress and the efficacy of anxiolytics: a new avenue of research, Physiology and Behavior, 73:337–342.

Hart, G., R. Copeland, 2010, Glycomics hits the big time, Cell, 143:672–676.

Hartl, D., A. Clark, 1997, Principles of population genetics, Sinaur Associates, Sunderland, MA.

Hazewinkel, M., 2002, Encyclopedia of Mathematics, 'Index Formulas', Springer, New York.

Hecht, M., A. Das, A. Go, L. Aradley, Y. Wei, 2004, *De novo* proteins from designed combinatorial libraries, Protein Science, 13:1711–1723.

Heine, S., 2001, Self as cultural product: an examination of East Asian and North American selves, Journal of Personality, 69:881–906.

Henrich J., S. Heine, A. Norenzayan, 2010, The weirdest people in the world? Behavioral and Brain Sciences, 33:61–83.

Hill, J., H. Wyatt, G. Reed, J. Peters, 2003, Obesity and the environment: where do we go from here? Science, 266:853–858.

Holling, C., 1973, Resilience and stability of ecological systems, Annual Reviews of Ecological Systematics, 4:1–23.

Holling, C., 1992, Cross-scale morphology, geometry, and dynamics of ecosystems, Ecological Monographs, 62:447–502.

Horrobin, D., 2003, Modern biomedical research: an internally self-consistent universe with little contact with medical reality?, Nature Reviews: Drug Discovery, 2:151–154.

Houghton, C., 1975, Wreath products of groupoids, Journal of the London Mathematical Society, S2-10(2):179–188.

Ikeda, N., S. Watanabe, 1989, Stochastic Differential Equations and Diffusion Processes, Second Edition, North Holland Publishing, Amsterdam.

Ives, A., 1995, Measuring resilience in stochastic systems, Ecological Monographs, 65:217–233.

Jablonka, E., 2004, Epigenetic epidemiology, International Journal of Epidemiology, 33:929–935.

Jablonka, E., M. Lamb, 1995, Epigenetic Inheritance and Evolution: The Lamarckian Dimension, Oxford University Press, Oxford.

Jablonka, E., M. Lamb, 1998, Epigenetic inheritance in evolution, Journal of Evolutionary Biology, 11:159–183.

Jacobson J., S. Jacobson, 2002, Breast-feeding and gender as moderators of teratogenic effects on cognitive development, Neurotoxicological Teratology, 24:349–358.

Jaenisch, R., A. Bird, 2003, Epigenetic regulation of gene expression: how the genome integrates intrinsic and environmental signals, Nature Genetics Supplement, 33:245–254.

James, L., D. Tawfik, 2003, Conformational diversity and protein evolution – a 60-year old hypothesis revisited, TRENDS in Biochemical Sciences, 28:361–368.

Jeffery, C., 2005, Mass spectrometry and the search for moonlighting proteins, Mass Spectrometry Reviews, 24:772–782.

Jenkins, J., A. Kleinman, B. Good, 1990, Cross-cultural studies of depression. In Becker, J., A. Kleinman, (eds.), Advances in mood disorders: Theory and Research, L. Erlbaum, Los Angeles, pp. 67–99.

Johnson-Laird, P., F. Mancini, A. Gangemi, 2006, A hyper-emotion theory of psychological illnesses, Psychological Reviews, 113:822–841.

Kahraman, A., 2009, The geometry and physicochemistry of protein binding sites and ligands and their detection in electron density maps, PhD dissertation, Cambridge University.

Karlin, S., H. Taylor, 1975, A First Course in Stochastic Pricesses, Second Edition, Academic Press, New York.

Karp, R., C. Chen, A. Meyers, 2005, The appearance of discretionary income: influence on the prevalence of under- and over-nutrition, International Journal of Equity in Health, 4:10.

Kastner, M., 2006, Phase transitions and configuration space, arXiv/cond-mat/0703401.

Kawaguchi, M., H. Mino, D. Durand, 2011, Stochastic resonance can enhance information transmission in neural networks, IEEE Transactions on Biomedical Engineering, 58:(7), doi 10.1109/TBME.2011.2126571.

Khinchin, A., 1957, The Mathematical Foundations of Information Theory, Dover, New York.

Kim, H., D. Sherman, S. Taylor, J. Sasaki, C. Ryu, J. Xu, 2010, Culture, serotonin receptor polymorphism (5-HTR1A) and locus of attention, Social, Cognitive, and Affective Neurosciences, 5:212–218.

Kim, J., R. Stewart, S. Kim, 2007, Interactions between life stressors and susceptibility genes (5-HTTLPR and BDNF) on depression in Korean elders, Biological Psychiatry, 62:423–428.

Kim, W., M. Hecht, 2006, Generic hydrophobic residues are sufficient to promote aggregation of the Alzheimer's $A\beta 42$ peptide, Proceedings of the National Academy of Sciences, 103:15824–15829.

Kitano, H., 2004, Biological robustness, Nature Reviews Genetics, 5:826–837.

Kivipelto, M., 2001, Midlife vascular risk factors for Alzheimer's disease in later life: longitudinal, population based study, British Medical Journal, 322:1447–1451.

Kleinman, A., B. Good, 1985, Culture and Depression: Studies in the Anthropology of Cross-Cultural Psychiatry of Affect and Depression, University of California Press, Berkeley.

Kleinman, A., V. Das, M. Lock, 1994, Social Suffering, University of California Press, Berkeley.

Kleinman, A., A. Cohen, 1997, Psychiatry's global challenge, Scientific American, 276(3):86–89.

Koonin, E., T. Senkevich, V. Dolja, 2006, The ancient virus world and evolution of cells, Biology Direct, 1:29.

Kung, Y., N. Ando, T. Doukov, L. Blasiak, G. Bender, J. Seravalli, S. Ragsdale, C. Drennan, 2012, Visualizing molecular juggling within a B_{12}-dependent methyltransferase complex, Nature, 484:265–269.

Kuo, W., Y. Chiang, T. Hwang, A. Wu, 2007, Performance-driven crosstalk elimination at postcompiler level – the case of low-crosstalk op-code assignment, IEEE Transactions on Computer-Aided Design of Integrated Circuits and Systems, 26:564–573.

Landau, L., E. Lifshitz, 2007, Statistical Physics, Part I, Elsevier, New York.

Landsteiner, K., 1936, The Specificity of Serological Reactions, reprinted 1962, Dover Publications, New York.

Langer, N., 1999, Culturally competent professionals in therapeutic alliances enhance patient compliance, Journal of Health Care for the Poor and Unverserviced, 10:19–26.

Lazarou, J., B. Pomeranz, P. Correy, 1998, Incidence of adverse drug reactions in hospitalized patients – a meta-analysis of prospective studies, Journal of the American Medical Association, 279:1200–1205.

Lei, J., K. Huang, 2010, Protein folding: a perspective from statistical physics, arXiv:1002.5013v1.

Levin, S., 1989, Ecology in theory and application. In Levin, S., T. Hallam, L. Gross (eds.), Applied Mathematical Ecology, Biomathematics Texts 18, Springer, New York.

Levinthal, C., 1968, Are there pathways for protein folding? Journal de Chimie Physique et de Physicochimie Biologique, 65:44–45.

Levinthal, C., 1969. In Debrunner, P., J. Tsbris, E. Munck (eds.) Mossbauer Spectroscopy in Biological Systems, University of Illinois Press, Urbana, pp. 22–24.

Levitt, M., C. Chothia, 1976, Structural patterns in globular proteins, Nature, 261:552–557.

Lewontin R., 2000, The Triple Helix: Gene, Organism, and Environment, Harvard University Press, Cambridge, MA.

Lewontin, R., 2010, Not so natural selection, New York Review of Books Online, May 27. http://www.nybooks.com/articles/archives/2010/may/ 27/not-so-natural-selection/?pagination=false

Littman, B., R. Krishna, 2011, Translational Medicine and Drug Discovery, Cambridge University Press, Cambridge.

Longuet-Higgins, H., 1963, The symmetry groups of non-rigid molecules, Molecular Physics, 6:445–460.

Luchinsky, D., 1997, On the nature of large fluctuations in equilibrium systems: observations of an optimal force, Journal of Physics A, 30:L577–L583.

Manolio, T., F. Collins, N. Cox, 2009, Finding the missing heritability of complex diseases, Nature, 461:747–753.

Manson, S., 1995, Culture and major depression: current challenges in the diagnosis of mood disorders, Psychiatric Clinics of North America, 18:487–501.

Marincola, F., 2011, The trouble with translational medicine, Journal of Internal Medicine, 270:123–127.

Markus H., S. Kitayama, 1991, Culture and the self: implications for cognition, emotion, and motivation, Psychological Review, 98:224–253.

Marsella, A., 2003, Cultural aspects of depressive experience and disorders. In Lonner, W., D. Dinnel, S, Hays, and D. Sattler (eds.), Online Readings in Psychology and Culture (Unit 9, Chapter 4) (http://www.wwu.edu/ culture), Center for Cross-Cultural Research, Western Washington University, Bellingham.

Masuda T., R. Nisbett, 2006, Culture and change blindness, Cognitive Science: A Multidisciplinary Journal, 30:381–399.

Matsumoto, Y., 2002, An Introduction to Morse Theory, American Mathematical Society, Providence.

Maturana, H., F. Varela, 1980, Autopoiesis and Cognition, Reidel Publishing Company, Dordrecht.

Maturana, H., F. Varela, 1992, The Tree of Knowledge, Shambhala Publications, Boston.

McCauley, J., 1993, Chaos, Dynamics and Fractals: An Algorithmic Approach to Deterministic Chaos, Cambridge University Press, New York.

Memmi, A., 1967, The Colonizer and the Colonized, Beacon Press, Boston.

Memmi, A., 1969, Dominated Man, Beacon Press, Boston.

Meyer, P., 1989, A short presentation on stochastic calculus. In Emery, M., Stochastic Calculus on Manifolds, Springer, New York.

Mian, I., C. Rose, 2011, Communication theory and multicellular biology, Integrative Biology, 3:350–367.

Miranda, M., D. Kim, M. Overstreet Galeano, C. Paul, A. Hull, S. Morgan. 2007. The relationship between early childhood blood lead levels and performance on end-of-grade tests, Environmental Health Perspectives, 115:1242–1247.

Miura, T., R. Kojima, M. Mizutani, Y. Shiga, F. Takatsu, Y. Suzuki, 2001, Effect of digioxin noncompliance on hospitalization and mortality in patients with heart failure in long-term therapy: a prospective cohort study, European Journal of Clinical Pharmacology, 57:77–83.

Modiano D., V. Petrarca, B. Sirma, I. Nebie, D. Diallo, F. Esposito M. Coluzzi, 1996, Different response to *Plasmodium falciparum* malaria in West African sympatric ethnic groups, Proceedings of the National Academy of Sciences, 93:13206–13211.

Modiano D., G. Luoni, B. Sirima, A. Lanfrancotti, V. Petrarca, F. Cruciani, J. Simpore, B. Ciminelli, E. Foglietta, P. Grisanti, I. Bianco, G. Modiano M. Coluzzi, 2001a, The lower susceptibility to *Plasmodium falciparum* malaria of Fulani of Burkina Faso (West Africa) is associated with low frequencies of classic malaria-resistance genes, Transactions of the Royal Society of Tropical Hygiene and Medicine, 95:149–152.

Modiano D., G. Luoni, V. Petrarca, B. Sodiomon Sirima, M. De Luca, J. Simpore, M. Coluzzi, J. Bodmer, G. Modiano, 2001b, HLA class I in three West African ethnic groups: genetic distances from sub-Saharan and Caucasoid populations, Tissue Antigen, 57:128–137.

Modiano D., V. Petrarca, B. Sirma, I. Nebie, G. Luoni, F. Esposito M. Coluzzi, 1998, Baseline immunity of the population and impact of insecticide-treated curtains on malaria infection, American Journal of Tropical and Medical Hygiene, 59:336–340.

Needleman, H., J. Riess, M. Tobin, G. Biesecker, J. Greenhouse, 1996, Bone lead levels and delinquent behavior, Journal of the American Medical Association, 275:363–369.

Nesse, R., 2000, Is depression an adaptation?, Archives of General Psychiatry, 57:14–20.

Nisbett R., K. Peng, C. Incheol, A. Norenzayan, 2001, Culture and systems of thought: holistic vs. analytic cognition, Psychological Review, 108:291–310.

Nocedal, J., S. Wright, 1999, Numerical Optimization, Springer, New York.

Norenzayan, A., S. Heine, 2005, Psychological universals: what are they and how can we know? Psychological Bulletin, 131:763–784.

Nunney, L., 1999, Lineage selection and the evolution of multistage carcinogenesis, Proceedings of the Royal Society B, 266:493–498.

Odling-Smee, F., K. Laland, M. Feldman, 2003, Niche Construction: The Neglected Process in Evolution, Princeton University Press, Princeton.

Ofria, C., C. Adami, T. Collier, 2003, Selective pressures on genomes in molecular evolution, Journal of Theoretical Biology, 222:477–483.

Onsager, L., S. Machlup, 1953, Fluctuations and irreversible processes, Physical Review, 91:1505–1512.

O'Nuallain, S., 2008, Code and context in gene expression, cognition, and consciousness. In Barbiere, M., (ed.), The Codes of Life: The Rules of Macroevolution, Springer, New York, pp. 347–356.

Onuchic, J., P. Wolynes, 2004, Theory of protein folding, Current Opinion in Structural Biology, 14:70–75.

Orr, G., R. Rando, F. Wen Bangerter, 1979, Synthetic glycolipids and the lectin-mediated aggregation of liposomes, Journal of Biological Chemistry, 254:4721–4725.

Oyelaran, O., Q. Li, D. Farnsworth, J. Gildersleeve, 2009, Microarrays with varying carbohydrate density reveal distinct subpopulations of serum antibodies, Journal of Proteome Research, 8:3529–3538.

Park, J., P. Neelakanta, 1996, Information-theoretic aspects of neural stochastic resonance, Complex Systems, 10:55–71.

Patterson, P., 2010, The trouble with multi-core, IEEE Spectrum, July: 28–53.

Paul, C., 1992, Introduction to Electromagnetic Compatibility, John Wiley and Sons, New York.

Paul, S., D. Mytelka, C. Dunwiddie, C. Persinger, B. Munos, S. Lindborg, A. Schact, 2010, How to improve R & D productivity: the pharmaceutical industry's grand challenge, Nature Reviews: Drug Discovery, 9:201–214.

Pauling, L., 1940, A theory of the structure and process of formation of antibodies, Journal of the American Chemical Society, 62:2643–2657.

Petersen, K., Ergodic Theory, Cambridge Studies in Advanced Mathematics 2, Cambridge University Press, New York.

Pettini, M., 2007, Geometry and Topology in Hamiltonian Dynamics and Statistical Mechanics, Springer, New York.

Pielou, E., 1977, Mathematical Ecology, Wiley, New York.

Pirmohamed, M., D. Naisbitt, F. Gordon, B. Park, 2002, The danger hypothesis – a potential role in idiosyncratic drug reaction, Toxicology, 181–182:55–63.

Plaxco, K., K. Simons, D. Baker, 1998, Contact order, transition state placement and the refolding rates of single domain proteins, Journal of Molecular Biology, 277:985–994.

Protter, P., 1990, Stochastic Integration and Differential Equations: A New Approach, Springer, New York.

Pufall, M., G. Lee, M. Nelson, H. Kang, A Velyvis, L. Kay, L. McIntosh, B. Graves, 2005, Variable control of Ets-1 DNA binding, Science, 309:142–145.

Qiu, C., M. Kivipelto, E. von Strauss, 2009, Epidemiology of Alzheimer's disease: occurrence, determinants, and strategies toward intervention, Dialogues in Clinical Neuroscience, 11:111–128.

Rau, H., T. Elbert, 2001, Psychophysiology of arterial baroreceptors and the etiology of hypertension, Biological Psychology, 57:179–201.

Richerson, P., R. Boyd, 2006, Not by genes alone: How Culture Transformed Human Evolution, University of Chicago Press, Chicago.

Ridley, M., 1996, Evolution, Second Edition, Blackwell Science, Oxford University Press, Oxford.

Ringle, G., J. Young, 1968, Solutions of the Heawood map-coloring problem, Proceedings of the National Academy of Sciences, 60:438–445.

Risch, N., R. Herrell, T. Lehner, K. Liang, L. Eaves, J. Hoh, A. Griem, M. Kovacs, J. Ott, K.R. Merikangas, 2009, Interaction between the serotonin transporter gene (5-HTTLPR), stressful life events, and risk of depression, Journal of the American Medical Association, 301:2462–2472.

Rockafellar, R., 1970, Convex Analysis, Princeton University Press, Princeton.

Rodin S., A. Rodin, 2008, On the origin of the genetic code: signatures of its primordial complementarity in tRNAs and aminoacyl-tRNA synthetases, Heredity, 100:341–355.

Royden, H., 1968, Real Analysis, Macmillan, New York.

Rudin, W., 1976, Principles of Mathematical Analysis, McGraw-Hill, New York.

Sackett, D., R. Haynes (eds.), 1976, Compliance with Therapeutic Regimens, Johns Hopkins University Press, Baltimore.

Sarlio-Lahteenkorva, S., E. Lahelma, 2001, Food insecurity is associated with past and present economic disadvantage and body mass index, Journal of Nutrition, 131:2880–2884.

Scherrer, K., J. Jost, 2007a, The gene and the genon concept: a functional and information-theoretic analysis, Molecular Systems Biology, 3:87–93.

Scherrer, K., J. Jost, 2007b, Gene and genon concept: coding versus regulation, Theory in Bioscience, 126:65–113.

Scheuner, D., R. Kaufman, 2008, The unfolded protein response: a pathway that links insulin demand with β-cell failure and diabetes, Endocrine Reviews, 29:317–333.

Shankardass, K., McConnell, R., Jerrett, M., Milam, J., Richardson, J., Berhane, K., 2009, Parental stress increases the effect of traffic-related air pollution on childhood asthma incidence, Proceedings of the National Academy of Sciences, 106:12406–12411.

Shannon, C., 1959, Coding theorems for a discrete source with a fidelity criterion, Institute of Radio Engineers International Convention Record Vol. 7, 142–163.

Shirkov, D., V. Kovalev, 2001, The Bogoliubov renormalization group and solution symmetry in mathematical physics, Physics Reports, 352:219–249.

Siliani, G., U. Frith, J. Demonet, F. Fazio, D. Perani, C. Price, C. Frith, E. Paulesu, 2005, Brain abnormalities underlying altered activation in dyslexia: a vowel based morphometry study, Brain, 128(Pt.10):2453–2461.

Sims-Robinson, S., B. Kim, A. Rosko, E. Feldman, 2010, How does diabetes accelerate Alzherimer's disease pathology? Nature Reviews Neurology, 6:551–559.

Singh-Manoux A., N. Adler, M. Marmot, 2003, Subjective social status: its determinants and its association with measures of ill-health in the Whitehall II study, Social Science and Medicine, 56:1321–1333.

Spenser, J., 2010, The giant component: the golden anniversary, Notices of the AMS, 57:720–724.

Stern, Y., 2009, Cognitive reserve, Neuropsychologica, 47:2010–2028.

Strauss, R., H. Pollack, 2001, Epidemic increase in chilhood overweight, 1986–1998, Journal of the American Medical Association, 286:2845–2848.

Sun, F., G. Ceataeno-Anolles, 2008, Evolutionary patterns in the sequence and structure of transfer RNA: a window into early translation and the genetic code, PLOSone, 3:32799.

Taylor, J., 1996, Introduction to Measure and Probability, Springer, New York.

Thayer, J., R. Lane, 2000, A model of neurovisceral integration in emotion regulation and dysregulation, Journal of Affective Disorders, 61:201–216.

Thomas K., 2012, J & J fined $1.2 billion in drug case, NY Times, April 12, B1-2.

Tlusty, T., 2007, A model for the emergence of the genetic code as a transition in a noisy information channel, Journal of Theoretical Biology, 249:331–342.

Tlusty, T., 2008, A simple model for the evolution of molecular codes driven by the interplay of accuracy, diversity and cost, Physical Biology, 5:016001.

Tlusty, T., 2008, Casting polymer nets to optimize noisy molecular codes, Proceedings of the National Academy of Sciences, 105:8238–8243.

Tlusty, T., 2010, Personal communication.

Tompa, P., P. Csermely, 2004, The role of structural disorder in the function of RNA and protein chaperones, FASEB Journal, 18:1169–1175.

Tompa, P., M. Fuxreiter, 2008, Fuzzy complexes: polymorphism and structural disorder in protein-protein interactions, Trends in Biochemical Science, 33:1–8.

Tompa, P., C. Szasz, L. Buday, 2005, Structural disorder throws new light on moonlighting, Trends in Biochemical Sciences, 30:484–489.

Turner, B., 2000, Histone acetylation and an epigenetic code, Bioessays, 22:836–845.

Ullmann, J., 1988, The Anatomy of Industrial Decline, Greenwood-Quorum Books, Westport.

Uversky, V., 2002, Natively unfolded proteins: a point where biology waits for physics, Protein Science, 11:739–756.

Vetsigian, K., C. Wose, N. Goldenfield, 2006, Collective evolution and the genetic code, Proceedings of the National Academy of Sciences, 103:10696–10701.

Villalobos, M., A. Mizuno, B. Dahl, N. Kemmotsu, R. Muller, 2005, Reduced functional connectivity between VI and Inferior frontal cortex associated with visimoto performance in autism, Neuroimage, 25:916–925.

Volkman, B. 2001, Two-state allosteric behavior in a single-domain signaling protein, Science, 291:2429-2433.

Wallace, D., 2001, Discriminatory public policies and the New York City tuberculosis epidemic, Microbes and Infection, 3:515–524.

Wallace, D., R. Wallace, 1998, A Plague on Your Houses, Verso, New York.

Wallace, D., R. Wallace, 1998, Scales of geography, time, and population: the study of violence as a public health problem, American Journal of Public Health, 88:1853–1858.

Wallace, D., R. Wallace, 2000, Life and death in Upper Manhattan and the Bronx: toward evolutionary perspectives on catastrophic social change, Environment and Planning A, 32:1245–1266.

Wallace, D., R. Wallace, V. Rauh, 2003, Community stress, demoralization, and body mass index: evidence for social signal transduction, Social Science and Medicine, 56:2467–2478.

Wallace, R., 2000, Language and coherent neural amplification in hierarchical systems: renormalization and the dual information source of a generalized spatiotemporal stochastic resonance, International Journal of Bifurcation and Chaos, 10:493–502.

Wallace, R., 2004, Comorbidity and anticomorbidity; autocognitive developmental disorders of psychosocial stress, Acta Biotheoretica, 52:71–93.

Wallace, R., 2005, Consciousness: A Mathematical Treatment of the Global Neuronal Workspace Model, Springer, New York.

Wallace, R., 2007, Culture and inattentional blindness: a global workspace perspective, Journal of Theoretical Biology, 245:378–390.

Wallace, R., 2008, Toward formal models of biologically inspired, highly parallel machine cognition, International Journal of Parallel, Emergent, and Distributed Systems, 23:367–408.

Wallace, R., 2009a, Metabolic constraints on the eukaryotic transition, Origins of Life and Evolution of Biospheres, 39:165–176.

Wallace, R., 2009b, Programming coevolutionary machines: the emerging conundrum, International Journal of Parallel, Emergent, and Distributed Systems, 24:443–453.

Wallace, R., 2010a, Protein folding disorders: toward a basic biological paradigm, Journal of Theoretical Biology, 267:582–594.

Wallace, R., 2010b, Tunable epigenetic catalysis: programming real-time cognitive machines, International Journal of Parallel, Emergent, and Distributed Systems, 25:209–222.

Wallace, R., 2011a, Structure and dynamics of the 'protein folding code' inferred using Tlusty's topological rate distortion approach, BioSystems, 103:18–26.

Wallace, R., 2011b, Multifunction moonlighting and intrinsically disordered proteins: information catalysis, non-rigid molecule symmetries and the 'logic gate' spectrum, Comptes Rendus Chimie, 14:1117–1121.

Wallace, R., 2011c, On the evolution of homochirality, Comptes Rendus Biologies, 334:263–268.

Wallace, R., 2012a, Extending Tlusty's rate distortion index theorem method to the glycome: do even 'low level' biochemical phenomena require sophisticated cognitive paradigms?, BioSystems, 107:145–152.

Wallace, R., 2012b, Spontaneous symmetry breaking in a non-rigid molecule approach to intrinsically disordered proteins, Molecular BioSystems, 8:374–377.

Wallace, R., 2012c, Consciousness, crosstalk, and the mereological fallacy: an evolutionary perspective, Physics of Life Reviews, doi 10.1016/j.plrev.2012.08.002.

Wallace, R., D. Wallace, J. Ullmann, H. Andrews, 1999, Deindustrialization, inner-city decay and the diffusion of AIDS in the USA, Environment and Planning A, 31:113–139.

Wallace, R., D. Wallace, 2005, Structured psychosocial stress and the US obesity epidemic, Journal of Biological Systems, 13:363–384.

Wallace, R., R.G. Wallace, D. Wallace, 2003, Toward cultural oncology: the evolutionary information dynamics of cancer, Open Systems and Information Dynamics, 10:159–181.

Wallace, R., M. Fullilove, 2008, Collective Consciousness and its Discontents, Springer, New York.

Wallace, R., D. Wallace, 1997, Community marginalization and the diffusion of disease and disorder in the United States, British Medical Journal, 314:1341–1345.

Wallace, R., D. Wallace, 2008, Punctuated equilibrium in statistical models of generalized coevolutionary resilience: how sudden ecosystem transitions can entrain both phenotype expression and Darwinian selection, Transactions on Computational Systems Biology IX, LNBI 5121:23–85.

Wallace, R., D. Wallace, 2009, Code, context, and epigenetic catalysis in gene expression, Transactions on Computational Systems Biology XI, LNBI 5750, 283–334.

Wallace, R., D. Wallace, 2010, Gene Expression and its Discontents: The Social Production of Chronic Disease, Springer, New York.

Wallace, R., D. Wallace, 2011, Cultural epigenetics: on the heritability of complex diseases, Transactions on Computational Systems Biology XIII, LNBI 6575:131–170.

Wallace, R., R. G. Wallace, 2008, On the spectrum of prebiotic chemical systems: an information-theoretic treatment of Eigen's Paradox, Origins of Life and Evolution of Bioshperes, 38:419–455.

Wallace, R.G., R. Wallace, 2009, Evolutionary radiation and the spectrum of consciousness, Consciousness and Cognition, 18:160–167.

Wallach, J., and M. Rey, 2009, A socioeconomic analysis of obesity and diabetes in New York City, Public Health Research, Practice, and Policy, Centers for Disease Control and Prevention, http://www.cdc.gov/pcd/issues/2009/jul/08_0215.htm.

Ward, L., 2009, Physics of neural synchronation mediated by stochastic resonance, Contemporary Physics, 50:563–574.

Weinstein, A., 1996, Groupoids: unifying internal and external symmetry, Notices of the American Mathematical Association, 43:744–752.

Wehling, M., 2011, Drug development in the light of translational science: shine or shade? Drug Discovery Today, 16:1076–1083.

West-Eberhard, M., 2003, Developmental Placisticity and Evolution, Oxford University Press, New York.

West-Eberhard, M., 2005, Developmental plasticity and the origin of species differences, Proceedings of the National Academy of Sciences, 102:6543–6549.

Wilkinson, R., 1996, Unhealthy Societies: The Afflictions of Inequality, Routledge, New York.

Wilson, K., 1971, Renormalization group and critical phenomena. I Renormalization group and the Kadanoff scaling picture, Physical Review B, 4:3174–3183.

Witzany, G., 2009, Noncoding RNAs: persistent viral agents as modular tools for cellular needs, Annals of the New York Academy of Sciences, 1178:244–267.

Wolpert, D., W. MacReady, 1995, No free lunch theorems for search, Santa Fe Institute, SFI-TR-02-010.

Wolpert, D., W. MacReady, 1997, No free lunch theorems for optimization, IEEE Transactions on Evolutionary Computation, 1:67–82.

Wolynes, P., 1996, Symmetry and the energy landscapes of biomolecules, Proceedings of the National Academcy of Sciences, 93:14249–14255.

Wymer, C., 1997, Structural nonlinear continuous-time models in econometrics, Macroeconomic Dynamics, 1:518–548.

Zhang, Q., Y. Wang, E. Huang, 2009, Changes in racial/ethnic disparities in the prevalence of type 2 diabetes by obesity level among US adults, Ethnicity and Health, 14:439–457.

Zhu, R., A. Rebirio, D. Salahub, S. Kaufmann, 2007, Studying genetic regulatory networks at the molecular level: delayed reaction stochastic models, Journal of Theoretical Biology, 246:725–745.

Index

adaptive landscape, 58
adiabatic, 10
adverse drug reactions, 153
aerobic transition, 48
Alzheimer's disease, 78, 168
animal consciousness, 7

benign neglect, 162
biological psychiatry, 67
biological renormalization, 115
blood pressure regulation, 14

cardiovascular disease, 78
channel capacity, 26, 35
coarse-graining, 50
codons, 83
coevolution, 37
coevolutionary system, 31
cognitive reserve, 173
convexity, 36
correlation length, 44
critical value, 115
crosstalk, 7
cultural environment, 66

differential reproduction, 47
diffusion paths, 31
DSM-IV, 63

ecological domain, 167
ecosystem resilience, 80
eigenmode, 146

eigenstate, 139
emotion, 14
endoplasmic reticulum, 78
environmental interaction, 49
epigenetic, 48, 67
epimutation, 73
ergodic, 10
evolutionary game dynamics, 57

felony convictions, 174
folding funnel, 77
free energy duality, 25
Fulani, 157

Gaussian channel, 26
gene expression, 15, 72
gene methylation, 48
generalized retina, 138
genetic heritage, 53
genomic complexity, 54
Gibbs distribution, 42
Glasperlenspiel, 4
global broadcast, 21
global workspace, 7
glycan determinants, 103
glycan spectra, 111
glycome, 15
glycomics, 99
grossly complicated topological
    object, 104
groupoid, 11, 196
groupoid representations, 82

Hamilton–Jacobi equation, 206
Hamiltonian, 29, 206
heredity, 47
hominid evolution, 16
HPA axis, 13, 144
human cognome, 11

idiotypic, 153
idiotypic network, 138
immune system, 8, 11
immunological homunculus, 137
index theorem, 32, 109, 125
internal self-image, 138
intrinsically disordered protein, 16
inverse Moore's Law, 1
irreducible representations, 82

Kuhn–Tucker optimization, 41, 151

Lagrange multiplier, 41, 151
Lambert W function, 22
large deviations, 31, 58, 204
lectin, 15, 116

magic bullet, 5
magic strategy, 6
malaria, 157
manufacturing job loss, 162
Markov assumption, 52
Martingale, 189
Martingale transform, 191
mass unemployment, 162
mental disorders, 63
mesoscale, 52
microreversibility, 29
missing heritability of complex
    diseases, 64
modern synthesis, 47
Morse function, 43, 86
mutation, 47

nearly ergodic process, 10
no free lunch theorem, 19
noise, 6
nonorthogonal, 139
nonrigid molecule, 122

obesity, 78
obesity epidemic, 160
ongoing activity, 9
optimization, 41
order parameter, 81, 115

pattern recognition, 9
percent unemployed, 168
percent unionized, 168
pharmaceutical research, 1
phenotype, 41
power law, 13
protein folding, 77
protein folding regulation, 15
protein symmetries, 102
pseudo probability, 124
psychological universals, 66
psychosocial stress, 138, 142, 144, 176

random networks, 20
rate distortion entropy, 36
rate distortion theorem, 84
real time, 35, 38
renormalization, 22, 115
resilience, 48
right-to-work, 170
rust belt, 162

sensory signal, 9
Shannon uncertainty, 10
signal transduction, 172
signal-to-noise ratio, 172
social capital, 162
social reality, 65
sociocultural network, 16
spandrel, 8, 20, 179
splitting criterion, 29
spontaneous symmetry breaking, 81
stationary, 10
stereochemistry, 124
stochastic differential equation, 30,
    189, 192
stochastic resonance, 6
symbolic dynamics, 50, 130
symmetry entropy, 125

therapeutic alliance, 143
topological decomposition, 102
topological hypothesis, 30
transitive groupoid, 196
translational medicine, 1
tumor control, 13
tunable catalyst, 90
type 2 diabetes, 77

typical sequences, 27

variation, 47
viral descent, 49

young elderly, 168

zero reference state, 139

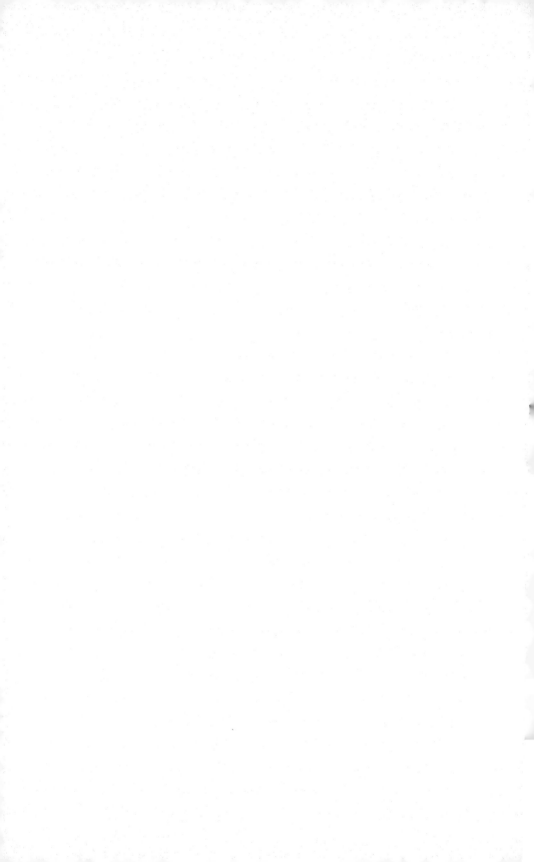